PROSTHODONTICS
at a Glance

PROSTHODONTICS
at a Glance

Sabita M Ram BDS MDS
Professor, Dean and Head
Department of Prosthodontics
Mahatma Gandhi Mission's Dental College and Hospital
Navi Mumbai, Maharashtra, India

Co-authors

Tulika Khanna BDS MDS
Reader
Department of Prosthodontics
Mahatma Gandhi Mission's Dental College and Hospital
Navi Mumbai, Maharashtra, India

Janani Iyer BDS MDS
Reader
Department of Prosthodontics
Mahatma Gandhi Mission's Dental College and Hospital
Navi Mumbai, Maharashtra, India

JAYPEE *The Health Sciences Publisher*

New Delhi | London | Panama

Jaypee Brothers Medical Publishers (P) Ltd

Headquarters
Jaypee Brothers Medical Publishers (P) Ltd.
4838/24, Ansari Road, Daryaganj
New Delhi 110 002, India
Phone: +91-11-43574357
Fax: +91-11-43574314
E-mail: jaypee@jaypeebrothers.com

Overseas Offices
J.P. Medical Ltd.
83, Victoria Street, London
SW1H 0HW (UK)
Phone: +44-20 3170 8910
Fax: +44(0)20 3008 6180
E-mail: info@jpmedpub.com

Jaypee-Highlights Medical Publishers Inc.
City of Knowledge, Bld. 235, 2nd Floor, Clayton
Panama City, Panama
Phone: +1 507-301-0496
Fax: +1 507-301-0499
E-mail: cservice@jphmedical.com

Jaypee Brothers Medical Publishers (P) Ltd.
17/1-B, Babar Road, Block-B, Shaymali
Mohammadpur, Dhaka-1207
Bangladesh
Mobile: +08801912003485
E-mail: jaypeedhaka@gmail.com

Jaypee Brothers Medical Publishers (P) Ltd.
Bhotahity, Kathmandu, Nepal
Phone: +977-9741283608
E-mail: kathmandu@jaypeebrothers.com

Website: www.jaypeebrothers.com
Website: www.jaypeedigital.com

Prosthodontics at a Glance

First Edition: **2018**

ISBN: 978-93-5270-098-1

Printed at Sanat Printers

Preface

Learning and appearing for exams is an integral part of the professional course. The subject of prosthodontics is being so vast that reading, remembering, comprehending and reproducing are seemed not easy. Additionally, phobia of the exam makes the student nervous and, at times, confused; not knowing from what to read to brush up his knowledge before facing a viva at the chairside exam.

A student is unable to go through all the books and revise the syllabus. However, he/she is looking for books to refresh, remember and reproduce knowledge.

A lot of things depend on how viva voce is faced and the precise manner in which the questions are answered. Students are looking forward to the information that is simple and easily remembered and reproduced.

This book has been written with the aim to help students recap their knowledge on the subject. Reading of the book will enable the students to confidently face the exam and answer the viva voce. It can be carried daily to the clinic for reference during chairside viva. It is a book which every student should posses as it will give answers to most of the question asked in prosthodontics. The book has been possible due to the inputs by our two staff members Dr Tulika Khanna and Dr Janani Iyer without their help it would not have been possible.

Special thanks to Shri Jitendar P Vij (Group Chairman), Mr Ankit Vij (Group President), Ms Ritu Sharma (Director-Content Strategy), and the whole team of M/s Jaypee Brothers Medical Publishers (P) Ltd, New Delhi, for their constant support and cooperation.

Sabita M Ram

Contents

CHAPTER 1

How to Face Viva Voce

How to Face Viva Voce

A viva is essentially a precise but detailed conversation with the student. It follows a fairly structured pattern. The time, place, length, participants and subject matter are established well in advance and one participant controls the proceedings and contributes mainly questions and the other contributes mainly the answers.

It has become one of the most important criteria in any selection procedure. A written test provides only an idea about the knowledge possessed by the candidate but does not indicate personal traits, behavioral pattern, confidence level, etc. and so oral tests (viva voce) have become very important.

In a viva, the observation of verbal and nonverbal responses are the chief features. Under verbal responses comes the manner of speaking, accent, language and the knowledge, etc. whereas nonverbal responses includes movements, etc.

By its nature, the viva sets up an artificial and often daunting relationship between people. The participants have to adopt roles and are not equal partners. If you take part in a viva, then with a proper strategy and preparation you could shine and come out with flying colors. The examiner's role is to judge and the student's job is to present themselves in favorable light. Hence, the student must do justice to himself or herself.

For many people, the time before a viva is a nerve racking, adrenalin-pumping period. Try to put all that adrenalin to positive use. This means first of all adopt a positive attitude. The underlying strategy for success is to value yourself. The viva does not require you to take on the role of victim. It is a dialogue and you are an active participant.

You may be the best candidate, but that is no guarantee that you will be evaluated and assessed to be the best. It is the proper preparation and experience that will make you sell yourself as the best person. Begin by thinking how you can make your best impression on the examiner. Not that you should present yourself as being different from what you are but you can present yourself in a very positive way. Consider what examiner is likely to ask. A prompt and flowing answer will always be in good light. Know your strengths and do not miss out on the opportunity to exhibit your strong areas. Also know your weak areas and try and see how you can circumvent them. Remember that most of the questions in a viva lead from one question to another and so plan your answers so that you can lead to your strong areas and evade weak areas.

On the day of the viva, allow yourself plenty of time to get ready. Reach the place of viva well in time. Ensure that you are not flustered when you arrive for the viva. Do not feel nervous and make friendly conservation with other students to ease up the tension, if required. Before you speak, you will be seen. The appearance should indicate your grasp and hence, it helps to be neatly dressed. Make sure your clothes are comfortable to wear and suite to you. Remember that you want to make good impression and be careful not to distract the examiner.

First impressions are of paramount importance and so, follow the following points:

- Enter the viva hall gently and exchange greetings of the day
- Sit with slight forward learning posture; put your hands in a natural and comfortable position
- Maintain the body posture which should not be too stiff or too relaxed
- While replying, make eye contact
- Speak with a slight smile
- Keep your cool and remain self controlled
- Answer questions in a concise, distinct and normal accent
- Control hand, body and finger movements
- Maintain self confidence and exhibit self assured style
- Establish good rapport with the examiner
- Keep your sentences short to the point
- While ending your answer, it is recommended to drop the pitch of your voice on the last syllable of your final sentence. This will indicate to examiner that you have completed your answer.

You can usually predict at least a few of the broad topics that will be raised during the viva. But it is unwise to predict the exact questions that might be asked to you. The question and answers that you wrote down and practiced with a friend should be no more than a rough guide.

Do not learn these answers by heart, as you run the risk of answering the wrong question. By all means prepare your ideas but not the exact words for conveying them. You could often find some difficult questions, those you hoped were never asked. Do not panic, pause, think and take your time to answer. Examiner is not looking for glib answers to difficult questions.

If the question is complicated and you do not understand, do not feel ashamed to ask the examiner to repeat the question. Do not allow yourself to be overwhelmed. Do not undersell yourself by giving up the difficult question without first trying to answer it. However, if you are really stuck and cannot answer then do not try to invent an answer. A quite confident admission of ignorance is more impressive than a bluster.

During a viva one must avoid the following points:

- Do not slam the door while entering the viva room. Avoid leaning back during the viva
- Do not fold arms or legs
- Avoid speaking in whispers or hushed tone or artificial accent
- Do not lose patience and get involved in an argument during the viva
- Do not remain too reserved or too arrogant
- Do not giggle or mumble during the viva
- Do not scratch yourself during the viva
- Do not tell lie and if you do not know the answer, say so
- Do not bite nails during the viva
- Do not launch into an answer without taking time to assemble your thoughts
- Do not think that you have to keep on talking until you are interrupted
- Do not talk in the abstract. Use specific examples
- Do not be too apologetic and in turn undersell yourself
- Do not exaggerate yourself or your knowledge.

At times, the examiner may ask you if you have any question at the end of the viva. In case you do wish to ask, ensure that it is constructive and in a positive spirit. You could then exhibit your initiative and imagination as well as knowledge and enthusiasm.

At the end of the viva, exchange greetings of the day and leave with a smiling face.

Summary

In short, day by day viva is becoming an important mode of evaluating capabilities. To be able to come out successful in viva, one must prepare oneself. For effective performance during the viva, one must be well studied in the subject, be present in time, neatly dressed, polite, alert, well-mannered and take time to reply and be positive in one's replies. One should not be nervous, self conscious and scared.

CHAPTER

2

Complete Dentures

Q. 1. Define prosthetic dentistry.

Ans. Prosthetic dentistry is that branch of dentistry pertaining to the restoration and maintenance of oral function, comfort, appearance and health of the patient by the restoration of natural teeth and/or the replacement of missing teeth and craniofacial tissues with artificial substitutes.

Q. 2. What is the aim of prosthetic dentistry?

Ans. The aim of prosthetic dentistry is restoration of missing or lost dentition and associated structures with a view to preserve what remains of the masticating apparatus, restore function and esthetics.

Q. 3. What are the objectives of prosthetic dentistry?

Ans. The objectives of prosthetic dentistry are:

- Elimination of oral disease to the greatest extent possible and patient's health
- Preservation of health and relationships of the teeth and health of oral and paraoral structures (facial appearance)

- Restoration of oral functions with esthetically pleasing end results.

Q. 4. What are the branches of prosthetic dentistry?

Ans. The branches of prosthetic dentistry are:

- **Removal prosthodontics:**
  Complete dentures
  Partial dentures
  Complete overdentures
  Partial overdentures.
- **Fixed prosthodontics:**
  Crowns
  Bridges
  Laminates.
- **Maxillofacial prosthodontics:**
  Obturators
  Stents
  Splints
  Extraoral prosthesis—eye,ear,nose,etc.
- **Implant prosthodontics:**
  Removable prosthesis
  Fixed prosthesis.

Q. 5. Define removable prosthodontics.

Ans. According to Glossary: It is that branch of Prosthodontics concerned with the replacement of teeth and contiguous structures for edentulous or partially edentulous patients by artificial substitutes that are removable from the mouth.

Q. 6. Define fixed prosthodontics.

Ans. According to Glossary, it is that branch of prosthodontics concerned with the replacement and/or restoration of teeth by artificial substitutes that are not readily removed from the mouth.

Q. 7. Define implant prosthodontics.

Ans. According to Glossary, it is that phase of prosthodontics concerning the replacement of missing teeth and/or associated structures by restorations that are attached to dental implants.

Q. 8. Define maxillofacial prosthodontics.

Ans. According to Glossary, it is that branch of prosthodontics concerned with the restoration and/or replacement of the stomatognathic and craniofacial structures with prosthesis that may or may not be removed on regular or elective basis.

Q. 9. Define complete dentures.

Ans. A dental prosthesis which replaces the entire dentition and associated structures of the maxilla and mandible.

Q. 10. Name the surfaces of a complete denture.

Ans. The surfaces of a complete denture are:

- **Polished surfaces:** Contoured as to support and contact the cheeks, lips and tongue
- **Impression or basal surfaces:** Fitted to basal seat area
- **Occlusal surfaces:** Occlusal surfaces of the teeth.

Q. 11. What are the functions of a complete denture?

Ans. Complete denture functions are to restore esthetics, mastication and phonetics.

Q. 12. What is diagnosis?

Ans. Diagnosis is defined as determination of nature of disease—GPT.

Q. 13. What is treatment planning?

Ans. Treatment planning is defined as the sequence of procedures planned for the treatment of a patient after diagnosis—GPT.

Q. 14. What is Dr MM House classification of mental attitudes of patients?

Ans.
- **The philosophical patient:** This type of patient presents the best mental attitude for denture acceptance. The patient is rational, sensible, calm and composed. The patient desires dentures for the maintenance of health and appearance.
- **The exacting patient:** This kind of patient may have all good attributes of the philosophical patient; however, he may require extreme, care and patience on part of the dentist. This patient is methodical, presice and accurate and at times, makes several demands.
- **The indifferent patient:** This type of patient presents a questionable or unfavourable prognosis. He is apathetic and uninterested and lacks motivation. He pays no attention to instructions, will not cooperate and is prone to blame the dentist for his poor oral health.
- **The hysterical patient:** This kind of patient is emotionally unstable, excitable, excessively apprehensive and hypertensive. The prognosis is often unfavourable and additional professional help is required prior to and during the treatment.

Q. 15. Which are the primary stress bearing areas in the maxillary foundation?

Ans. Slopes of the residual ridge and most of the hard palate are the primary stress bearing areas in the maxillary foundation.

Q. 16. Which is the primary stress bearing area in the mandibular foundation?

Ans. Buccal shelf is the primary stress bearing area in the mandibular foundation.

Q. 17. Why the buccal shelf area is regarded as the primary stress bearing area in mandibular foundation?

Ans. The buccal shelf area consists of smooth compact cortical bone. Its position is at right angles to the occlusal forces and thus, it is selected as the primary stress bearing area.

Q. 18. What are the boundries of buccal shelf area?

Ans. Boundaries of buccal shelf area are:

- Medially: Crest of residual alveolar ridge.
- Anteriorly: Buccal frenum
- Laterally: External oblique ridge
- Distally: Retromolar pad.

Q. 19. What is retromylohyoid fossa and what are its boundries?

Ans. It is the area posterior to mylohyoid muscle. It extends from the end of the mylohyoid ridge to the retromylohycid curtain. This is also known as the lateral throat form and is bounded by:

Anteriorly	:	Mylohyoid muscle
Laterally	:	Pear shaped pad
Posterolaterally	:	Superior constrictor muscle
Medially	:	Tongue.

Q. 20. Name the secondary stress-bearing areas in the maxillary foundation.

Ans. The rugae and maxillary tuberosity are the secondary stress bearing areas in the maxillary foundation.

Q. 21. Name the secondary stress-bearing areas in the mandibular foundation.

Ans. Slopes of the residual alveolar ridge is the secondary stress bearing area in the mandibular foundation.

Q. 22. Which are the areas in the maxillary foundation that offer retention?

Ans. The areas in the maxillary foundation that offer retention are:

- Hard palate
- Residual alveolar ridge
- Rugae
- Peripheral tissues
- Posterior palatal seal area
- Undercuts, if present.

Q. 23. Which are the areas in the mandibular foundation that offer retention?

Ans. The areas in the mandibular foundation that offer retention are:

- Buccal shelf
- Residual ridge
- Peripheral tissues
- Undercuts.

Q. 24. Which are the relief areas in maxillary foundation?

Ans. The relief areas in maxillary foundation are:

- Median palatal suture and its overlying raphe
- Incisive papillae
- Torus palatinus (if present)
- Palatine rugae (if prominent).

Q. 25. Which are the relief areas in mandibular foundation?

Ans. The relief areas in mandibular foundation are:

- Crest of the residual alveolar ridge when it is sharp and thin
- Torus mandibularis
- Mental foramen
- Mylohyoid ridge
- Genial tubercles, if present.

Q. 26. How do you classify lateral throat form?

Ans. Neil classifies retromylohyoid fossa as:

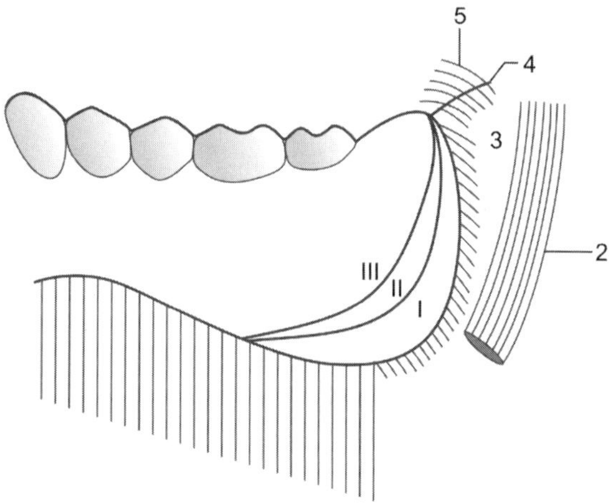

Class I: Class I throat form indicates that the anatomical structures will accommodate a fairly long and wide flange. The thickness varies greatly. The horizontal border is usually 2–3 mm thick, but a thicker border of 4–5 mm should be used for better seal, if the border is flat.

Class II: The class II lateral throat form is about half as long and narrow as the class I and about twice as long as class III.

Class III: A class III lateral throat form has minimum length and thickness. The border usually ends 2–3 mm below the mylohyoid ridge or sometimes just at the ridge. The thickness should be no more than approximately 2 mm; or, it may even end in a knife edge if the border terminates at the mylohyoid ridge.

Q. 27. What are genial tubercles?

Ans. According to Glossary, genial tubercles are mental spines. They are rounded elevations (usually 2 pairs) clustered around midline on the lingual surface of the lower portion of the mandibular symphysis. These tubercles serve as attachments for the genioglossus and geniohyoid muscles.

Q. 28. When are the genial tubercles visible?

Ans. Genial tubercles are visible when there is a resorbed mandibular foundation.

Q. 29. Should you cover the genial tubercle?

Ans. Yes, they should be covered in a resorbed mandible when they are visible. Seal in premylohyoid area can be achieved by placing the border seal beyond the genial tubercles by covering them.

Q. 30. Which muscles are associated with maxillary buccal frenum?

Ans. Orbicularis oris (anteriorly), buccinator (posteriorly) and caninus also called as levator anguli oris (vertically) are the three muscles associated with the maxillary buccal frenum.

Q. 31. What are the muscles in the labial frenum?

Ans. There are no muscles in the labial frenum. It is only a fold of mucous membrane.

Q. 32. Which muscles dictate the buccal flange of maxillary and mandibular dentures?

Ans. Buccinator and masseter are the muscles dictating the buccal flange of maxillary and mandibular dentures.

Q. 33. What are the contents of retromolar pad?

Ans. The contents of retromolar pad area are loose connective tissue, glandular tissue, and insertion of fibers of temporalis tendon posteriorly, buccinator fibers laterally and fibers of superior constrictor and pterygomandibular raphe medially.

Q. 34. What is the significance of the retromolar pad?

Ans. The significance of retromolar pad is that it determines the distal limit of mandibular denture and aids in the stability of denture by adding another plane to resist movement of the base. It also acts as a support area and does not resorb as it contains insertion of the muscles which have constant stimulation on it.

Q. 35. What is a maxillary torus? What is its significance?

Ans. Maxillary torus is a smooth rounded anatomical bony protuberance in the mid palatal area.

It is a relief area and if not relieved, acts as a fulcrum and leads to instability of the denture. It further causes ulceration and irritation of tissues overlying the torus. It may lead to fracture of denture in the midline.

Relief must be provided during the fabrication of denture at the final impression stage and the packing stage.

Q. 36. What is sublingual crescent area? What is its importance?

Ans. The anterior region of lingual sulcus is termed as sub-lingual crescent area. It is also termed as the premylohoid area.

The crescent shape is due to the presence of the sublingual salivary glands. The length and width of the border in this area is important in maintaining peripheral seal of lower denture.

Q. 37. What is posterior palatal seal area?

Ans. The soft tissues along the junction of the hard and soft palate on which pressure within physiologic limits of the tissues can be applied by a denture to aid in the retention of a denture.

Q. 38. How do you mark the posterior palatal seal in patients' mouth?

Ans. Patient is made to sit in upright position. With the help of T burnisher, hamular notch is located and marked with pencil. The line is extended 3-4 mm anterolaterally to mucogingival junction and do the same on opposite side. Ask the patient to say "ah" with short vigorous burst (sharry methods) to demarcate the anterior vibrating line. For drawing posterior vibrating line, patient is asked to say "ah" in short bursts in normal, unexaggerated manner.

Q. 39. What is posterior palatal seal?

Ans. It is the seal achieved between the posterior aspect of the denture and the nonmovable aspect of the soft palate.

Q. 40. Why the anterior vibrating line is cupid's bow in shape?

Ans. Anterior vibrating line is cupid's bow in shape because of the presence of posterior nasal spine.

Q. 41. How do you classify soft palate?

Ans. Ley's classification is based on angle of soft palate:

Class 1: Soft palate horizontal with minimum muscular activity and wide posterior palatal seal which is not deep.

Class 2: The angle of attachment lies between class 1 and 2.

Class 3: More acute contour in relation to hard palate. Seen in V shaped hard palate, it has small posterior palatal seal but it is deep.

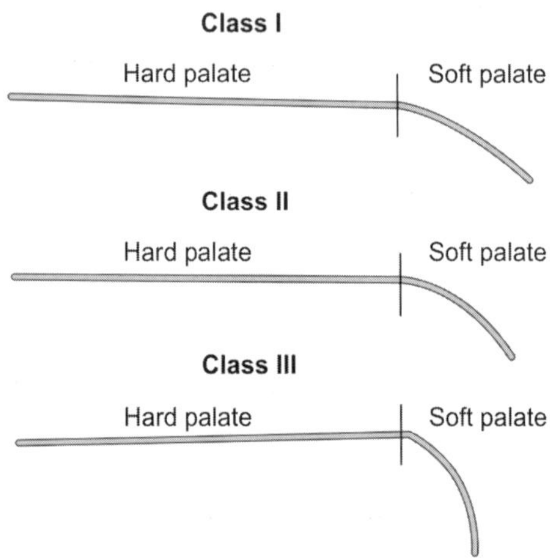

Classification by Bernard Levin:

Class 1: Greater than 5 mm movable tissue. Ideal for retention,usually thin denture base is advisable.

Class 2: 1–5 mm of movable tissue, good retention is usually possible, medium thickness of denture base is needed.

Class 3: Less than 1 mm of movable tissue, retention is poor, thick denture base is needed.

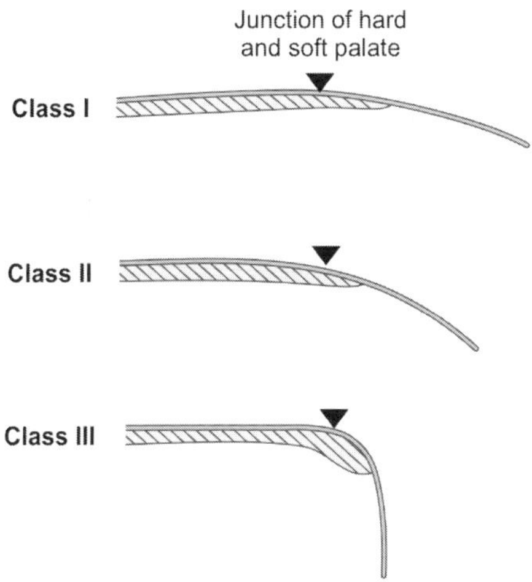

Q. 42. What is the purpose of posterior palatal seal?

Ans. The following are the purposes of posterior palatal seal area:

- Retention of maxillary denture
- Reduction in patient's awareness to denture
- Reduction in gag reflex
- Reduction in food accumulation beneath the denture
- Compensates for the volumetric shrinkage occurring during polymerization.

Q. 43. What are the different methods of obtaining posterior palatal seal?

Ans. The different methods of obtaining posterior palatal seal are:

- Conventional approach

- Fluid wax technique
- Arbitrary scraping of master cast
- Extended palatal technique by Silverman
- Modified technique-continuation with border-molding.

Q. 44. What is the anatomic boundaries of the posterior palatal seal area?

Ans. The posterior palatal seal extends medially from one tuberosity to the other. Laterally, the pterygomaxillary seal extends through the hamular notch continuing for 3–4 mm anteriolaterally approximating the mucogingival junction.

Q. 45. What are anterior and posterior vibrating lines?

Ans. Anterior vibrating line:

It is an imaginary line lying at the junction between the nonmovable tissues of the hard palate and slightly movable tissues of the soft palate.

Posterior vibrating line:

The imaginary line across the posterior part of the soft palate marking the division between the movable and nonmovable tissues of the soft palate. It is called as the AH line. This can be identified when the patient says "AH". It is beyond this imaginary line, the soft palate can be seen to move.

Q. 46. What are the problems, if the denture is placed beyond the posterior vibrating line?

Ans. The denture would be considered overextended leading to:

- Gagging
- Irritation of the soft palate tissues
- Loss of retention.

Q. 47. What is fovea palatinae?

Ans. They are opening in the posterior region of the palate, formed by coalescence of ducts of several palatal mucous salivary glands.

Q. 48. When and why should you locate the posterior palatal seal area?

Ans. The posterior palatal seal area, i.e. the posterior and anterior vibrating lines should be located at the primary impression stage.

Locating it at the primary impressions stage will help to fabricate the final impression tray which will extend accurately for recording the posterior palatal seal area at final impressions stage to achieve a proper seal.

Q. 49. When can you achieve posterior palatal seal?

Ans. The posterior palatal seal could be achieved at the following stages in a complete denture:

- Final impression stage
- Try-in stage
- Denture delivery stage.

Q. 50. What are the most important areas for achieving retention in maxillary denture?

Ans. The posterior palatal seal area and the coronomaxillary space are important areas for achieving a retentive maxillary denture.

Q. 51. What is coronomaxillary flange of the maxillary denture?

Ans. The coronomaxillary flange of the maxillary denture is that portion of the buccal flange that extends from the zygomatic eminence to the hamular notch.

Q. 52. How do you record coronomaxillary space?

Ans. The patient is asked to half open his mouth and move the mandible laterally. This brings the coronoid process closer to the maxillary tuberosity and thus, records the area in question.

Q. 53. What are the other names for coronomaxillary space?

Ans. The following terms have been used to identify the coronomaxillary space:

- Buccal space or vestibule
- Buccal pocket
- Tuberosity sulcus
- Distobuccal angle of the buccal vestibule
- Buccal sulcus
- Buccal pouch
- Buccal mucous membrane reflection region
- Postmalar area.

Q. 54. How will you record the massetric notch area while making mandibular impression?

Ans. The massetric notch is registered in the impression by the action of the anterior border of the masseter muscle. When recording the impression for the massetric notch patient should be asked to close his mouth against resistance. This will activate the anterior border of the masseter muscle and get registered as a notch in the impression.

Q. 55. Define impression in complete denture patients.

Ans. A complete denture impression is a negative registration of entire denture bearing, stabilizing and border seal areas present in the edentulous mouth which is recorded when the plastic material becomes relatively hard or set while in contact with the tissues.

Q. 56. What are the objectives of impression making?

Ans. The objectives of impression making are:

- To provide retention, stability and support for denture
- To act as foundation for improving esthetics
- To maintain health of the tissues and preserve them.

Q. 57. What are the purposes of primary impression?

Ans. The purposes of a primary impression are:

- Diagnosis and treatment planning
- Fabrication of a special tray/custom tray to make final impression.

Q. 58. What is the purpose of final impression?

Ans. The purpose of final impression is to make a cast which is used for fabrication of the complete denture so as to achieve retention, stability, support, esthetics and preservation of tissues.

Q. 59. What are the different impression techniques used in complete denture?

Ans. The different impression techniques used in complete denture are according to:

- **Mouth position**
  - Closed mouth technique
  - Open mouth technique.
- **Pressure exerted while impression making**
  - Pressure techniques (Green Brothers compound)
  - Minimum pressure technique (Harry L Page)
  - Selective pressure technique (Boucher et al.)
  - Modified techniques for flabby tissues, poor foundation and compromised ridges.

Q. 60. What are different theories of impression making?

Ans. Different theories of impression making are:

- Mucostatic
- Mucocompressive
- Selective pressure technique.

Q. 61. Who advocated the mucostatic impression technique?

Ans. Harry L Page advocated the mucostatic impression technique.

Q. 62. What materials can be used for making primary impression for completely edentulous patient?

Ans. The materials which can be used for making primary impressions for completely edentulous patient are:

- Medium fusing compound type I
- Putty (elastomeric impression materials)
- Irreversible hydrocolloids (alginates).

Q. 63. What are the advantages of using impression compound for making primary impression in complete denture patients?

Ans. The advantages of using impression compound as a primary impression material are:

- It can support itself in cases where the stock metal tray is short.
- It can be re-softened and impression can be repeated, if not properly recorded at the first instance.
- The primary impression made in impression compound can be used as a tray for making final impression.
- It has a good shelf life.

Q. 64. What are advantages of using irreversible hydrocolloids for making impressions in complete denture patients?

Ans. The advantages of using alginate for making primary impressions are:

- It does not require warm water bath unlike for impression compound.
- Easy to manipulate
- More comfortable for patients sensitive to heat
- Exerts less pressure
- It can be used in case of bilateral undercuts.

Q. 65. What is the temperature of water used for manipulating impression compound during primary impression making?

Ans. The temperature of water should be 60–70°C for manipulating impression compound during primary impression making.

Q. 66. What happens, if the temperature of the water bath used for manipulating compound is above 70°C?

Ans. The plasticisers from the impression compound leach out hampering the workability. This may also cause mucosal burns.

Q. 67. What is the importance of border molding?

Ans. Border molding records the peripheral tissues by slightly displacing them to achieve a seal and make effective the factor of atmospheric pressure to achieve retention.

Q. 68. Define border molding.

Ans. The shaping of the border areas of an impression by functional or manual manipulation of the tissue adjacent to the border to duplicate the contour and the size of the vestibule.

Q. 69. What is peripheral seal?

Ans. Peripheral seal is the contact of the denture border with the underlying or adjacent tissues, it prevent the passage of air or other substances beneath the denture. It is also known as border seal.

Q. 70. After you achieve peripheral seal, which factor of retention comes into play?

Ans. Atmospheric pressure comes into play once peripheral seal has been established.

Q. 71. What are the materials used for border molding?

Ans. The materials used for border molding are:

- Low fusing compound
- Metallic pastes (zinc oxide eugenol/noneugenol impression paste) thick consistency
- Elastomers–putty consistency
- Mouth temperature waxes
- Autopolymerizing acrylic resin.

Q. 72. What are the different forms of low fusing compound sticks?

Ans. Low fusing compound are available in variety of colors like green, brown, gray, black and white.

Q. 73. What are the materials used for making a final impression in complete denture?

Ans.

- Impression plaster
- Metallic pastes (zinc oxide eugenol/non-eugenol impression paste)

- Elastomers—medium or light body
- Tissue conditioners
- Irreversible hydrocolloids (alginates) with adequate spacer
- Mouth temperature waxes eg. IOWA wax, Korrecta wax.

Q. 74. When would you indicate a pressure impression?

Ans. Pressure impression should never be indicated as it may give immediate retention but causes ischemia of the tissues leading to resorption of the bone and loss of retention.

Q. 75. Does minimum pressure impression technique use border molding?

Ans. Minimum pressure impression believes in the principle of recording the tissues with minimum pressure and the borders are kept short of the peripheries.

Retention is by adhesion, cohesion and interfacial surface tension.
No border molding is done.

Q. 76. When will you indicate a minimum pressure impression?

Ans. When peripheral tissues are not resilient, e.g. submucous fibrosis or scarring of tissues.

Q. 77. Define retention in complete dentures.

Ans. Retention in complete dentures is defined as the resistance to displacement of the denture base away from the ridge.

According to Glossary, retention is that quality inherent in the prosthesis which resists the forces of gravity, adhesiveness of food and the forces associated with the opening of the jaws.

Q. 78. Define stability in complete denture.

Ans. Stability is defined as the quality of a denture to be firm, steady, or constant, to resist displacement by functional stresses and not to be subjected for change of position when forces are applied.

Q. 79. Define support in complete denture.

Ans. Support is the resistance of a denture to the vertical force of mastication, occlusal forces and other forces applied in a direction toward the denture bearing area.

Q. 80. Name the factors that affect retention in complete denture.

Ans. The factors that affect retention in complete denture are:

- **Physical factors:**
  - Adhesion and cohesion
  - Interfacial surface tension
  - Capillary attraction
  - Atmospheric pressure
  - Gravity.
- **Antomical factors:**
  - Size of denture bearing area
  - Quality of denture bearing area
  - Resiliency of peripherial tissues.
- **Physiological factors:**
  - Saliva
  - Consistency of saliva
  - Quantity of saliva.
- **Muscular factors:**
  - Neuromuscular control

  - Forces of buccal musculature
  - Forces of the tongue.
- **Mechanical factors:**
  - Undercuts
  - Implants
  - Springs
  - Magnets
  - Denture adhesive.

Q. 81. Name the factors of stability in complete dentures?

Ans. The factors of stability are:

- The relationship of the denture base to the underlying tissues (impression surface)—surface area, closeness of contact, height of residual ridge
- The relationship of the external surface and border to the surrounding orofacial musculature (polished surface)
- The relationship of the opposing occlusal surfaces (occlusal surface)
  - Occlusal plane parallel to the ridge
  - Form and position of the teeth.

Q. 82. Name the factors of support in complete dentures.

Ans. The factors of support are the following:

- Coverage the occlussal factors to stress bearing areas and relieving the nonstress-bearing areas
- Confining the occussal forces to stress bearing areas and relieving the nonstress-bearing areas.

Q. 83. Name different types of jaw relation records.

Ans. Different types of jaw relations records are:

- Orientation relation
- Vertical relation
- Horizontal relation.

Q. 84. What is the importance of orientation relation?

Ans. The importance of orientation relation is that it orients the maxilla and the mandible in relation to the hinge axis and base of skull. It records the position of the jaws in three dimension and transfer this to an articulator to stimulate jaw position.

Q. 85. Define orientation relation.

Ans. According to Glossary, the jaw relation when the mandible is kept in its most posterior position, it can rotate in the sagittal plane around an imaginary transverse axis passing through or near the condyles.

Q. 86. How will you adjust the maxillary occlusal rim at the jaw relation stage?

Ans.

- Check for lip support
- Check for visibility, i.e. length of the rim
  - Normal lip length: 1–2 mm visibility
  - Short lip length: Visibility more than 2 mm
  - Long lip length: No visibility.
- Check the parallelism of the rim.
  - Anteriorly parallel to interpupillary.
  - Posteriorly parallel to ala tragus line.
- Check the space availability between the maxillary rim and mandibular ridge.

If space is inadequate, compensate maxillary rim to provide space for mandibular rim.

Q. 87. What is a face bow?

Ans. Face bow is a caliper like device that is used to record the relationship of the jaws to the TMJ, in turn, the face bow helps to relate, record and transfer the relationship of the maxilla to the hinge axis and transfer this relationship to the articulator as it exists in the patient.

According to Glossary, a caliper like device which is used to record the relationship of the maxilla and/or the mandible to the temporomandibular joints.

Q. 88. What is the significance of face bow?

Ans.
- Transverse hinge axis can be located with the aid of face bow.
- Records the position of maxilla in three planes with reference to cranium.
- To relate the maxillary casts to the transverse axis of the articulator.
- Mandibular hinge axis coincided and related to the maxillary by centric relation record.
- The path of closure will be similar.
- It aids in securing the anteroposterior cast position in relation to the condyles of the mandible.
- Failure to use face bow can lead to error in occlusion of denture.
- Facc bow transfer allows more accurate arc of closure on the articulator when the interocclusal records are used.

Q. 89. What are the different types of face bows?

Ans. Face bows are of two types:

1. Arbitrary face bows:
   - Fascia
   - Earpiece
   - Spring bow
   - Slidematic.
2. Kinematic face bow.

Q. 90. What are the various parts of face bow?

Ans. The parts of face bow are as follows:

U-shaped frame, bite-fork, orbital pointer, condylar rods, locking device.

Q. 91. What is hinge axis?

Ans. Hinge axis is the imaginary line around which the condyles can rotate without translation.

Q. 92. What is terminal hinge axis?

Ans. It is the most retruded hinge position around which the condyles can rotate without translation, it is learnable, repeatable and recordable position. It coincides with centric relation.

Q. 93. What are the differences between arbitrary and kinematic face bow?

Ans. Arbitrary face bow is placed on the face with condyle rods located approximately over the condyles. The rods are within 5 mm of the true center of the opening axis of the jaws. Whereas kinematic face bow helps to locate the true center of the condyle on which the condylar rods are positioned to take the face bow record.

Arbitrary face bow are generally used for edentulous patients while kinematic face bow are used for dentulous patients.

Q. 94. Write the commonly used anterior and posterior reference points.

Ans. Anterior reference points are as follows:

- Orbitale—It is the lowest point on the infraorbital rim along with the two posterior points forms the axis known as orbitale plane.
- Orbitale minus 7 mm—The anterior point of reference marked 7 mm below orbitale on the patient or 7 mm above orbital indicator.
- Nasion minus 23 mm
- Incisal edge plus articulator midpoint to articulator axis—horizontal plane distance

- Alae of the nose—In complete dentures, the tentative occlusal plane is made parallel with the horizontal plane.
- Posterior reference points are as follows:
- Beyron point—A point 13 mm anterior to the posterior margin of the tragus of ear on a line from the center of the tragus to the outer canthus of the eye.
- Bergstrom point—A point 10 mm anterior to the center of the spherical insert for the external auditory meatus and 7 mm below the Frankfort horizontal plane.

Q. 95. Define physiologic rest position of mandible.

Ans. Physiologic rest position of mandible is defined as the mandibular position assumed when the head is in an upright position and the involved muscles, particularly the elevator and depressor groups, are in equilibrium in tonic contraction and the condyles are in a neutral; unstrained position.

Q. 96. What are the different methods of determining vertical relation of occlusion?

Ans. The different methods of recording/determining vertical relation of occlusion are:

- Anatomical methods:
  - Preextraction
    - Cast in occlusion
    - Profile cut out
    - Profile photograph
    - Patient's mask
    - Tattoo method
    - Wright's method
    - Radiographic.

- Postextraction records
  - Equal 3rd method
  - Willi's distance method
  - Ridge relationship
  - Former dentures
  - Radiographic.
- Physiological methods:
  - Niswonger's method
  - Swallowing threshold method
  - Phonetics.
- Boos bimeter
- Electromyography
- Transcutaneous electrical nerve stimulation (TENS method).

Q. 97. What are the consequences of an increased vertical relation?

Ans. The consequences of an increased vertical relation are:

- Difficulty in speech and mastication
- More visibility of teeth, poor esthetics
- Pain under the basal seat of dentures and inflammation
- At later stage:
  Pain in temporomandibular joint (TMJ) and resorption of ridges.

Q. 98. What are the consequences of decreased vertical relation?

Ans. The consequences of a decreased vertical relation are:

- Less space for tongue—speech affected and pain in ear
- Poor esthetics; senile appearance
- Angular chelitis
- Pain in TMJ
- Decrease in masticatory efficiency.

Q. 99. Define centric relation.

Ans. According to Boucher, it is defined as the most posterior relation of the lower jaw to the upper jaw from which lateral movements can be made at a given vertical dimension.

According to Glossary of Prosthodontic, it is defined as the most retruded relation of the mandible to the maxilla when the condyles are in the most posterior unstrained position in the glenoid fossae from which the lateral movements can be made at any given degree of jaw separations.

The maxillomandibular relationship in which the condyles articulate with the thinnest avascular portion of their respective disks with the complex in the anterior-superior position against the shapes of the articular eminences. This position is independent of tooth contact. This position is clinically discernible when the mandible is directed superior and anteriorly. It is restricted to a purely rotary movement about the transverse horizontal axis (GPT 8).

Q. 100. What is the significance of centric relation in complete denture?

Ans. The significance of centric relation in complete denture are:

- It helps establish centric occlusion in edentulous patients.
- It is a comfortable position for the patient.
- It is a repeatable position.
- It is a readable position.

Q. 101. What are the different methods of recording centric relation?

Ans. The different methods of recording centric relation are:

- Static-check bite record
- Functional methods:
  - Patterson's chew-in-technique
  - Needle house technique
- Graphic methods
  - Intraoral tracing
  - Extraoral tracing
- Radiographic
- Hinge axis.

Q. 102. How will you guide your patient to close in centric relation?

Ans. To close in centric relation patient can be:

- Guided by the operator:
  - Chin point guidance (Goichet)
  - Bimanual method (Peter Dawson)
  - Three finger method (Peter Thomas).
- Assisted to retrude mandible:
  - Place the tip of the tongue on the posterior end of the palate and close
  - Bite on the posterior teeth
  - Place the lower jaw backward
  - Swallow and close
  - Bend the head forward or backwards.

Q. 103. What are the consequences of incorrectly recorded centric relation?

Ans. The consequences of incorrectly recorded centric relation are:

- Improper occlusion between mandibular and maxillary teeth; inability to masticate
- Instability and pain in the underlying tissues
- TMJ affected/discomfort; pain in TMJ
- Discomfort in parafunctional movements.

Q. 104. What are the different materials which can be used to prepare temporary record bases?

Ans. For temporary record bases materials used are:

- Shellac base plate
- Self cured acrylic resin
- Light cured resins
- Vaccum formed vinyl or polystyrene
- Hard wax.

Q. 105. What are materials used for permanent record bases?

Ans. For permanent record bases, the various materials used are:

- **Resin**
  Processed heat cured acrylic resin.
- **Metal**
  Base metal alloys, e.g. chromium-cobalt alloy and chromium-nickle alloy, and precious metals like gold. Combination of resin and metal.

Q. 106. What are the important points to be considered during jaw relations?

Ans. Stable—retentive and comfortable denture bases, denture bases relieved at all frenal attachments, smooth, well rounded denture borders.

Q. 107. What are the advantages and disadvantages of heat cured acrylic resin bases constructed for recording jaw relation?

Ans. Advantages of heat cured acrylic resin bases:

- Rigid
- Accurate
- Stable—no distortion
- Strength is good—not easily broken

- Retention, stability, support and esthetics can be assessed at the jaw relation stage.

Disadvantages of heat cured acrylic resin bases:

- Difficult to arrange the teeth
- Time consuming
- Loss of final cast
- Distortion of the base due to second curing.

Q. 108. What is the importance of the nick and notch while recording centric relation?

Ans. The nick prevents lateral or side movements while the notch prevents the anterior–posterior movement.

Q. 109. What is an articulator?

Ans. An articulator is a mechanical device which represents the temporomandibular joints and jaw members to which maxillary and mandibular casts may be attached to stimulate jaw movements.

Q. 110. What are the advantages of using an articulator?

Ans. Following are some of the advantages of articulator:

- Properly mounted casts allow the operator to better visualize the patients occlusion, especially from lingual view.
- Patient cooperation is not a factor when using an articulator. Once appropriate, interocclusal records are obtained from the patient.
- It reduces the chair time and patient appointment time.
- The refinement of complete denture occlusion in the mouth is extremely difficult because of shifting denture bases and resiliency of the supporting tissue.
- Interocclusal records can be obtained and complete denture occlusion can be refined outside the mouth on an articulator.

- More procedures can be delegated to auxillary personnel when utilizing an articulator for development of patient's occlusion.

Q. 111. How do you classify articulators?

Ans. Articulators can be classified as follows:

Based on theories of occlusion:

- Bonwill theory
- Conical theory
- Spherical theory.

Based on adjustability of articulator:

- Non-adjustable
  - Simple hinge
  - Hinge with fixed condylar control.
- Semi-adjustable
  - Arcon
  - Non-arcon—Hanau, Dentatus.
- Fully adjustable
  - Denar
  - TMJ.

Q. 112. What are acron and non-acron articulators?

Ans. Acron articulators are those which cont~ins the condylar path elements within its upper member and the condylar elements within the lower member. This instrument maintains anatomic guidelines by the use of condylar analogs in the mandibular element and fossae assemblies within the maxillary element. On the contrary, non-acron articulator contains condylar elements in its upper member.

Q. 113. What is the difference between a semi adjustable and fully adjustable articulator? Give one example of each.

Ans. The semi-adjustable articulator does not represent the exact movement of the condyles. The movements recorded are represented on the articulator in straight angles. It is not considered as the exact duplication of the movements of the patient's condyle.

Example: Hanau, Whipmix, Dentatus.

A full adjustable articulator can accept and reproduce the exact movements of the patient's TMJ. Example: Denar and TMJ articulator.

Q. 114. What is Bennett movement?

Ans. The bodily lateral movement or lateral shift of the mandible resulting from the movement of the condyles along the lateral inclines of the mandibular fossa in lateral movements. It was described by Dr Norman Bennett in 1985 and thus, called Bennett movement and Shift. The average side shift is 1.5–2 mm.

Q. 115. What is Bennett angle?

Ans. It is the angle at which the non-working condyle moves along the medial slope of glenoid fossa. The average Bennett angle is 12°.

Q. 116. What is tissue Realeff?

Ans. Hanau called it as "Tissue Realeff" the resiliency and like effects based on resiliency of the supporting soft tissues.The making of impressions, recording and verifying of jaw relations and harmonizing of the occlusion of teeth to coincide with jaw movements are greatly influenced by the quantity and quality of soft tissues.

Q. 117. What are the criteria for selection of anterior teeth?

Ans. The criteria for selection of anterior teeth is basically related to esthetics, should be in harmony with face and overall appearance of the patient.

They can be selected according to:

- **Size:**
  - Preextraction records-photographs, casts, X-rays
  - Anthropological measurements
    - ¤ Length - High lip line
    - ¤ Width - Canine line
    - ¤ Size of face

      1/16 of bizygomatic width = width of maxillary central incisor

      1/3rd of bizygomatic width = width of maxillary anteriors
    - ¤ Circumference of the head/10= width of maxillary central incisor
- **Shape and form:**
  - Form of patient face—square, tapered, ovoid
  - Dentogenic, sex, personality, age (SPA factor)
- **Shade:** Hue, chroma and value
- **Material:** Ceramic, resins or composite.

Q. 118. What are the criteria for selection of posterior teeth?

Ans. The criteria for selection of posterior teeth is basically related of function (mastication) and occlusion. They are:

- **Size:** Buccolingual—pounds triangle

  Mesiodistal—distal of the canine to the anterior of the retromolar pad or ascending slope of ramus
- **Form:**
  - Anatomic
  - Semi-anatomic
  - Non-anatomic—zero degree
- **Shade:** To match the anterior teeth
- **Materials:**
  - Ceramic

- Resin
- Composite
- Metal occlusal inserts.

Q. 119. How will preextraction records help in selection of anterior teeth?

Ans. Preextraction guides includes photographs, diagnostic casts and radiographs.

Q. 120. What is SPA factor in selection of anterior teeth?

Ans. Sex, personality, age is SPA factor in selection of anterior teeth.

Q. 121. What is dentogenic concept?

Ans. Frush and Fisher introduced the dentogenic concept for selection and arrangements of anterior teeth integrated towards system of esthetics. They advised dentist to choose, alter the form of teeth, arrange and contour gingiva to be in harmony with the patient's sex, personality and age.

Q. 122. What are different posterior tooth forms?

Ans. The different posterior tooth forms are:

- Anatomic—33°
- Semi anatomic—less than 20°
- Non-anatomic/monoplane/zero°.

Q. 123. What are the different materials used for posterior teeth?

Ans. The different materials used for posterior teeth are:

- Ceramic
- Acrylic resins
- Composite resins
- Metal inserts.

Q. 124. In which cases can you give posterior porcelain teeth?

Ans. Posterior Porcelain teeth can be given when adequate inter-ridge space exists and residual ridges are well-formed.

Q. 125. What are the advantages and disadvantages of using porcelain teeth?

Ans. **Advantages of porcelain teeth:**

- More resistant to abrasion
- Maintain lusture
- More esthetic
- Resistant to staining.

Disadvantages of porcelain teeth:

- Does not bond chemically to denture base
- Tend to chip and fracture
- Increased stress transmission to underlying tissues
- Chattering sound on occlusion.

Q. 126. What are the indications of using monoplane teeth?

Ans. Monoplane teeth are indicated in the following situations:

- In cross arch relationship of jaws
- Inability to record correct centric relation due to lack of neuromuscular coordination
- Poor or resorbed ridges
- Knife edge ridge.

Q. 127. What are the advantages and disadvantages of using monoplane teeth?

Ans. **Advantages:**

- Reduced vertical stresses
- Reduced horizontal stress due to absence of tooth incline

- Freedom in centric
- Reduced ridge resorption.

Disadvantages:

- Reduced masticatory efficiency
- Reduced esthetics
- Muscle fatigue.

Q. 128. How will you determine the mesiodistal width of posterior teeth?

Ans. The mesiodistal width of posterior teeth is determined by measuring the edentulous area between the distal of the mandibular canine and the ascending ramus of the mandible which is situated slightly anterior to the retromolar pad. The maxillary posteriors should occupy the space between the distal of the maxillary canine and the anterior of the tuberosity. No tooth should be placed on the retromolar pad or maxillary tuberosity.

Q. 129. How should you arrange the teeth buccolingually to favour the stability of mandibular denture?

Ans. The stability is enhanced when mandibular teeth are placed on the crest of the mandibular ridge or slightly lingual without encroaching on the tongue space.

Q. 130. What is buccal corridor?

Ans. It is a dark space between the buccal surface of the posterior teeth and the corner of the lips/cheek when the patient smiles.

Q. 131. What is the importance of the buccal corridor?

Ans. The buccal corridor affect the final esthetics. A large buccal corridor will have less teeth visiblity whereas a less buccal corridor will have more teeth visiblity. Large buccal corridor gives an elderly appearance.

However, less corridor will have a more toothy appearance.

Q. 132. What is occlusion?

Ans. The Glossary of Prosthodontic defines occlusion as "the relationship between the occlusal surfaces of the maxillary and mandibular teeth when they are in contact. It is a static position."

Q. 133. What is articulation?

Ans. Hanau used the term articulation to define the contacting of teeth as the mandible moved to and fro in centric relation or eccentric relation.

Q. 134. What are the differences between natural and artificial teeth?

Ans. The differences between natural and artificial teeth are as follows:

- In natural dentition, teeth are retained by periodontal tissues and when they are lost, both occlusion and proprioceptive feedback mechanisms are lost. In artificial occlusion, all teeth are arranged on the basis of soft tissues rest.
- In natural occlusion, teeth receive individual pressures of occlusion and can move independently. The artificial teeth move as a unit on their base.
- Malocclusion of natural teeth will effect individual teeth. Improper occlusion in dentures will effect the stability and position of the denture as a whole
- Incising with natural teeth does not effect posterior teeth, while in dentures it causes instability, when anterior teeth are used for incising.
- Bilateral balance is rarely found in natural dentition. In dentures, bilateral balance gives stability and comfort.

Q. 135. What are the different theories of occlusion in complete dentures?

Ans. The different theories of occlusion in complete denture are:

1. Balanced : Centric
Eccentric—lateral
protusive
2. Non-Balanced : Neutrocentric—centralization of occlusion, pitch, position, number
Organic—muscle and Joint without tooth function
Monoplane
Lingualized.

Q. 136. What is centric occlusion?

Ans. Centric occlusion is the relation of opposing occlusal surfaces that provides the maximum planned contact and/or intercuspation.

Q. 137. What is the difference between centric occlusion and centric relation?

Ans. Centric occlusion is a tooth-to-tooth relation, whereas centric relation is a static position and is a bone-to -bone relation.

Centric occlusion and centric elation may not coincide in natural dentition. However, centric occlusion and centric relation must coincide in artificial dentures. Thus, centric occlusion is established at the centric relation in artificial dentures.

Q. 138. Define balanced occlusion.

Ans. Balanced occlusion is defined as the stable simultaneous contacting of maxillary and mandibular teeth on the right and left, and in the anterior and posterior occlusal areas when the jaws are in either centric or eccentric relation.

Q. 139. What is balanced articulation?

Ans. It is the simultaneous contacting of the teeth as the mandible moves to and from the centric relation and eccentric relation.

Q. 140. What are the advantages of balanced occlusion?

Ans. The advantages of balanced occlusion are:

- Ensures even pressure on the ridges
- Prevents bone resorption due to even distribution of forces
- Maintain the stability of dentures when the mandible is in centric or eccentric positions
- Minimizes the lateral occlusal forces whereby maintaining stability
- Comfort to the patient in functional and parafunctional movements.

Q. 141. What are the factors of balanced occlusion?

Ans. The factors of balanced occlusion are:

- **Condylar guidance**—patient factor—not under control of the operator
- **Incisal guidance**—dictated by esthetics and phonetics—partially under control of the operator
- **Orientation of the plane of occlusion**
- Orientation of the plane of occlusion.
- Cuspal angulation
- Compensating curves

Q.142. Define Incisal guidance.

Ans. Incisal guidance is the influence of the contacting surfaces of the mandibular and maxillary anterior teeth on mandibular movements.

or

Incisal guidance is the influence of the contacting surfaces of the guide pin and guide table on articulator movements.

Q. 143. Define condylar guidance.

Ans. Condylar guidance by Glossary of prosthodontics is mandibular guidance generated by the condyle and articular disc traversing the contour of the glenoid fossae.

Or

Condylar guidance is the mechanical form located in the upper posterior region of an articulator that controls movement of its mobile member.

It is controlled By operator to achieve balanced occlusion.

Q. 144. What is the compensating curve?

Ans. The anterior—posterior curvature in the median plane and the mediolateral curvature in the frontal plane in the alignment of the occluding surfaces and the incisal edges of the artificial teeth that are used to develop balanced occlusion is known as compensating curve.

The curve introduced in the construction of complete denture to compensate for the opening influences produced by the condylar and the incisal guidance during lateral and protrusive mandibular excursive movements.

Q. 145. What is Monson's curve?

Ans. The lower natural teeth are inclined slightly to the lingual, which creates a transverse curve of occlusal surfaces from side to side. This is called Monson's curve, which has about an 8" diameter for normal dentition.

Q. 146. What is pleasure curve?

Ans. Pleasure or Anti Monson's curve is eponym for a helicoids curve of occlusion that, when viewed in frontal plane, conforms to a curve that is convex from the superior view except for last molars which reverse the pattern.

Or

Pleasure curve is reversal or occlusal plane of posterior teeth except 3rd molar whereby the occlusal surfaces of mandibular teeth slope facially instead of lingually and those of maxillary teeth incline lingually in excessive wear of teeth, obliteration of or formation of either flat or worn out occlusal surface.

Q. 147. How will a steep condylar guidance affect the compensating curve?

Ans. As the compensating curve is in harmony with movement of mandible as guided posteriorly by condylar path a steep condylar guidance will require a steep compensating curve for occlusal balance thereby affecting it.

Q. 148. What is Christensen's phenomenon?

Ans. The development of distal wedge shape spaces between the upper and lower occlusal surfaces of the occlusion rims or dentures in protusion is known as the Christensen phenomenon. It was first seen by Christensen. It is also seen in natural dentition. It is caused because of the downward and forward movement of the condyle.

Q. 149. Can Christensen's phenomenon be eliminated in complete denture construction? And how?

Ans. Yes, it can be eliminated by incorporating the compensating curve while arranging teeth.

Q. 150. How will you achieve balance with monoplane teeth?

Ans. Balance can be achieved with monoplane teeth by balancing ramp or tilting of mandibular last molars to contact the upper teeth in protrusion.

Q. 151. What are functional cusps?

Ans. The plunger cusps—the palatal cusp of the maxillary and buccal cusps of the mandibular are the functional cusps.

Q. 152. What is the purpose of a try-in in complete denture fabrication?

Ans. Try-in is important for the following purposes:

- To check for retention, stability, support of denture and comfort of the patient
- To verify the maxillomandibular records made at the time of jaw relations, i.e. centric and vertical relation
- To determine position of teeth and contours of denture base
- To evaluate esthetics
- To make interocclusal records, if needed
- To take patient's approval.

Q. 153. How will you check the vertical relation of occlusion at the try-in stage for your complete denture patient?

Ans. The vertical relation of occlusion at try-in stage can be checked by 5 methods. They are:

1. Check for the free way space—2–3 mm measure d by Niswonger method when patient is at vertical dimension of rest.

2. Check for the interocclusal space which should be more than the freeway space when the patient talks.
3. Check for the position of the lower anterior teeth. They should be at the lower lip.
4. Check for the Silverman's speaking space—1mm between the maxillary and mandibular incisors when patient says "S".
5. Esthetic—Evaluation of overall esthetics. Patient's face should not give too full or over closed appearance.

Q. 154. If at try-in appointment stage, an error is observed in the centric relation, how will you correct it?

Ans. An error observed in centric relation at try-in appointment can be corrected by removing the lower posterior teeth and recording centric relation by placing softened wax on the lower posterior region and asking the patient to close on the back teeth thus, impressing the cusps of the opposing teeth into wax at the desired vertical dimension of occlusion.

Even if one side intercuspation is not perfect, teeth on both side right and left should be removed to record the centric relation again.

Q. 155. What is free way space?

Ans. Freeway space is the distance between the occluding surfaces of maxillary and mandibular teeth when the mandible is in its physiologic rest position. It helps us to arrive at the vertical dimension of occlusion. The difference of the vertical dimension of rest and vertical dimension of occlusion will give the free way space.

Q. 156. What is Silverman's closest speaking space?

Ans. Silverman's closest speaking space is defined as the closest relationship of incisal edges of the mandibular teeth to the maxillary teethe during function, rapid speech or when patient says "S" it is 1–2 mm. It was first described by Silverman.

Q. 157. What is the importance of horizontal overlap [overjet] and vertical overlap [overbite]?

Ans. Horizontal overlap and vertical overlap help in esthetics, speech and achieving balanced occlusion.

When the overbite is increased, the overjet also requires to be increased, if not done will lead to interference and instability of dentures. The nonanatomic posterior teeth when arranged in monoplane occlusion do not require a vertical but horizontal overlap should be given.

Q. 158. In which stage should you pack the heat cure acrylic into the mould?

Ans. The heat cure acrylic is packed in dough stage.

Q. 159. Why do you apply cold mold (sodium alginate) seal to the dewaxed mould?

Ans. It is applied as a separating medium to form a layer between the plaster and acrylic resin. Reaction of sodium alginate and plaster forms calcium alginate which acts as a separating film between plaster and resin.

Q. 160. What are the curing cycles for the heat cure acrylic resin?

Ans. There are two curing for heat cure acrylic resin. They are:

1. Long curing cycle: 60°–70°C for 9 hours

2. Short curing cycle: 65°C for 90 minutes then 100°C for 60 minutes.

Q. 161. What are the advantages of metallic denture bases?

Ans. The advantages of metallic denture bases are:

- Thermal conductivity
- More strength in thinner sections
- Dimensional stability
- Increased tissue tolerance
- Increased retention and stability
- Reduced bulk with better function of speech.

Q. 162. What are the disadvantages of metallic denture bases?

Ans. The disadvantages of metallic denture bases are:

- Inability to be rebased or relined
- Poor esthetic qualities
- High cost.

Q. 163. Why is internal porosity seen in thick sections of dentures?

Ans. Internal porosity is seen in thick sections of dentures when exothermic heat cannot be dissipated through the plaster, the temperature in the thick portion of the acrylic resin may rise above the boiling point of monomer (100.8°C) causing porosity.

Q. 164. What are the other causes of porosity?

Ans. The other causes of porosity are:

- Improper mixing of resin; too much monomer
- Exposure of the resin while manipulation, allowing the monomer to evaporate
- Packing at the stingy stage
- Underpacking of resin, lack of pressure while packing of polymerization

- Improper curing
- Curing at very high temperature.

Q. 165. What is laboratory remount?

Ans. It is mounting of deflasked dentures on the parent articulator to check for the processing errors in occlusion. These errors can be eliminated by carrying out the selective grinding.

Q. 166. What is selective grinding?

Ans. The intentional alteration of the occlusal surfaces of teeth to change their form, to achieve the desired occlusion.

Q. 167. In selective grinding, which cusps should you avoid grinding?

Ans. In selective grinding, the cusps that we should avoid grinding are the functional cusps. They are:

- Maxillary—lingual cusps
- Mandibular—buccal cusp.

Q. 168. What is patient remount?

Ans. Patient remount is to remount the dentures on an articulator by means of interocclusal records made in the patient's mouth at the time of denture insertion or later. This is done to over come the effects of tissue resilency.

It could also be done if occusal interferences are detected which are gross and can not be eliminated at the chairside.

Q. 169. What instructions will you give to a patient at the time of denture insertion?

Ans. Instructions to be given to patient at time of insertion are:

- Adjustment care sequence
  - 1st appointment within 24 hours of delivery is must.
  - 2nd appointment after 4 days, if patient complains of pain or discomfort.
  - 3rd appointment after 1 week following 2nd adjustment.
  - If patient experiences problems, they must see the dentist.
- For the first 24 hours, the denture should be worn in the night for the patient to adjust and adapt to them
  - After the 1st appointment, patient should be instructed to remove the denture at night.
  - When dentures are taken out of the mouth they should be kept in water in a container with a tight lid.
  - Denture should not be dipped in or cleaned with warm water.
- Cleaning of dentures
  - Denture should be cleaned after every meal by rinsing with water.
  - Denture should be cleaned with brush and liquid detergent once a day.
  - Denture should be cleaned with a denture cleaning powder or tablets once a week by soaking dentures overnight for removal of stains, e. g. Clensodent, Steradent, Fitty Dent.
- Food intake and mastication
  - Patient should take in small morsels of food
  - Should chew on both sides
  - Should avoid extremely hard and sticky food
  - Should avoid incising with front teeth.

- Talking
  - Should be told to read aloud
  - Sip water occasionally while talking.
- Repair
  - Patient should be instructed not to repair dentures, if broken with feviquick or gums, etc. but visit the dentist immediately.
- Renewal of denture
  - Patient should have new dentures fabricated after the 3rd year or earlier, if the dentures are ill fitting or teeth have worn out.

Q. 170. Which is the chemical used in the denture cleaning powder?

Ans. Sodium perborate monohydrate is the chemical used in the denture cleaning powder. This liberates nascent oxygen which helps to remove stains and clean dentures.

Q. 171. What are the causes of food accumulating under denture?

Ans. Causes of food accumulating under denture are:

- Improper peripherial seal
- Occlusal interference
- Chewing only on one side
- Under-extension of denture borders.

Q. 172. What are the causes of gagging in new patient with complete denture?

Ans. Causes of gagging in new patient with complete denture are:

- Over-extension of the maxillary denture
- Inadequate posterior palatal seal
- Thick denture in the posterior palatal seal area

- Over-extension of the mandibular denture in the retromylohyoid area
- Reduced vertical dimension of occlusion
- Large tongue.

Q. 173. How will you reduce gagging at various stages of denture fabrication?

Ans.
- Instruct the patient to rinse with chilled water prior to impression making. Try and distract the patients attention by engaging him in conversation.
- Apply a topical anesthetic agent on the palate, if required.
- At impression stage, avoid overfilling the impression tray, make the primary impression with impression compound as it does not flow down the throat.
- Proper extension and placement of posterior palatal seal is required.
- Maintain the correct vertical dimension of occlusion, a low vertical will cause the tongue to fall back and trigger the gag reflex.
- At denture delivery stage, instruct the patient to wear only the upper denture for the first day. Once he is able to tolerate one denture, he should wear the other and should alternate the dentures until he is comfortable, only then should he be instructed to wear both the dentures.

Q. 174. What are the causes of cheek-bite?

Ans. The causes of cheek-bite are:

- Insufficient horizontal overlap of posterior teeth
- In case of very laxed buccal musculature
- Reduced vertical height.

Q. 175. What are the causes of inefficiency in chewing?

Ans. The causes of inefficiency in chewing are:

- Nonanatomic posterior teeth
- Lack of interdigitation of posterior teeth
- Use of acrylic teeth in a patient who is earlier used to porcelain teeth
- Locked occlusion or unbalanced occlusion
- Low vertical dimension of occlusion
- Incorrect centric relation.

Q. 176. What is the difference between relining and rebasing?

Ans. Relining is a process of resurfacing tissue surface of a denture with new base material to make it fit more accurately. While rebasing is a process of replacing the entire denture base material with new material.

Q. 177. When is relining indicated?

Ans. The indication for relining is when there is resorption of the ridge and dentures lack retention and stability. It is for refitting of the impression surface.

Q. 178. When is relining contraindicated?

Ans.

- Worn out dentures
- Vertical dimension loss greater than 7 mm
- Significant mucosal inflammation
- Poor denture esthetics
- Denture related speech problems
- Severe tooth wear
- Vertical overlap with tooth wear (posterior tooth concept)
- Severe occlusal wear (complete denture evaluation).

Q. 179. When is rebasing indicated?

Ans. Rebasing is indicated when there is:

- Discoloration of denture base
- Porosity of denture base.

Q. 180. What are soft liners?

Ans. They are elastomer polymers used in the prevention of chronic soreness from denture and the preservation of supporting structures.

The vinyl and acrylic polymers are made resilient by the addition of only an alcohol type plasticizers or by co- polymerization with the monomer unit. The hydrophilic polymer is a mixture of polyethylene glycol with diacetins.

Q. 181. What are the indications and contraindications of use of soft liners?

Ans. The indications of use of soft liners are:

- Ridge atrophy or resorption
  - Bruxers
  - Surgery.
- The contraindications of use of soft liners are:
  - Relief areas
  - Xerostomia
  - Obturators to enhance retention
  - Dentures opposing natural dentition.

Q. 182. What are tissue conditioners?

Ans. Tissue conditioners are composed of polyethyl-methacrylate or one of its copolymers and a mixture of aromatic ester and ethyl alchohol. These are advocated to rehabilitate inflammed and abused tissues, prior to making impressions.

Q. 183. What is the difference between soft liners and tissue conditioners?

Ans. Tissue conditioners are indicated to condition the abused tissue. Soft liners are indicated to give a cushioning effect to relieve and project vulnerable tissues.

Q. 184. What are the major uses of tissues conditioners?

Ans. They are used for:

- Tissue treatment
- Temporary obturators
- Base plate stabilization
- Liners in surgical splints
- Trial denture base
- Functional impression material.

Q. 185. What are transitional denture and their advantages?

Ans. Transitional dentures are removable partial dentures serving as an interim prosthesis to which artificial teeth can be added when natural teeth are lost or extracted.

The various advantages are as follows:

- Help to prepare patient to accept prosthesis
- Psychological benefit
- Esthetics.

Q. 186. Define over dentures and write their advantages.

Ans. A removable partial denture or complete denture that covers and rest on one or more remaining natural teeth, the roots of natural teeth and/or dental implants is called over denture.

The various advantages are as follows:

- Preservation of alveolar bone
- Periodontal maintenance

- Preservation of properioceptive response
- Support
- Retention
- Patient acceptance
- Convertibility to complete dentures
- Harmony of arch form.

Q. 187. What are the disadvantages of overdentures?

Ans. Disadvantages of over dentures are:

- Caries susceptibility
- Bony undercuts prevent close approximation of the denture flange to underlying tissue
- Over contoured dentures
- Under contoured dentures
- Encroachment of interocclusal distance
- Periodontal breakdown of a abutment teeth.

Q. 188. What is an immediate denture?

Ans. An immediate denture is a complete or removable partial denture fabricated for placement immediately following the removal of natural teeth. It is fabricated prior to the extraction of teeth and placed immediately after extraction.

Q. 189. What are the indications for immediate dentures?

Ans. The indications include patients with periodontally weak teeth indicated for extraction but patients cannot go through the edentulous period without dentures due to social, psychological and personal needs.

Q. 190. What are the advantages of immediate dentures?

Ans. The advantages of immediate dentures are:

- Psychological benefit to the patient, he does not have to appear edentulous at any point of time.

- Muscle tone, tongue size and vertical dimension are preserved.
- Centric jaw relation is easy to record.
- Less postoperative pain, because the extraction sockets are protected by the denture.
- Postoperative hemorrhage and infection are prevented due to the denture.
- Tooth size, shape, shade selection and arrangement are easy.
- It is easier for the patient to adapt to the permanent prosthesis.

Q. 191. What are the disadvantages of immediate dentures?

Ans. The disadvantages of immediate dentures are:

- They require more chair side time
- They are more expensive
- If prematurities in occlusion are present, recording centric relation is difficult
- Anterior try-in is not possible.

Q. 192. Classify cleft palate.

Ans. Classification of cleft palate by Veau:

Class 1 : Involving soft palate only

Class 2 : Involving soft and hard palate up to incisive foramen.

Class 3 : Involving soft and hard palates through alveolar ridge and continued into lip on one side.

Class 4 : Involving both soft and hard palates with bilateral cleft-lip.

Q. 193. What is an obturator?

Ans. Obturator is a prosthesis used to close a congential or acquired tissue opening, primarily of the hard palate and/or contiguous alveolar structures. Prosthetic restoration of the defeat often includes use of surgical obturator, in term obturator and definitive obturator.

Q. 194. What are the different types of obturators?

Ans. The different types of obturators are as follows:

- **For congential defects**
  - Feeding plates
  - Speech appliance
  - Overlay or superimposed denture
  - Bulb obturator.
    - ¤ Fixed - fixed
    - ¤ Hinge
    - ¤ Meatal
- **For acquired Defeats**
  - Surgical/treatment obturator
  - Interim—obturator
  - Definitive obturator

Q. 195. Define implant dentistry.

Ans. Implant dentistry is the selection, planning, development, placement and maintenance of restoration using dental implants.

Q. 196. What is an implant denture?

Ans. A denture which receives its support, stability and retention from a substructure which is partially or wholly implanted under the soft tissues of the denture basal seat.

Q. 197. What is a dental implant?

Ans. A prosthetic device of alloplastic material (s) implanted into the oral tissues beneath the mucosal and/or periosteal layer, and on/or within the bone to provide retention and support for a fixed or removable prosthesis; a substance that is placed into and/or upon the jaw bone to support a fixed or removable prosthesis.

Q. 198. What are the different parts of implants?

Ans. Fixture, abutment, abutment screw and crown. These are the parts of implant.

Q. 199. Classify dental implants based on their anchorage component as it relates to the alveolar bone?

Ans. According to the relation of anchorage component of dental implant to the alveolar bone, the dental implants can be;

- Mucosal
- Endosteal or endosseous
- Transsosseous
- Sub periosteal
- Endodontic.

Q. 200. What are the various forms of implants?

Ans. The various forms of implants are:-

- Button shaped—mucosal implants
- Blade—endosteal or endosseous
- Cylindrical, smooth or threaded—endosteal or endosseous.
  - Solid
  - Hollow
  - Partial hollow—corevent
- Root form endosteal or endosseous
- Screw form endosteal or endosseous
- Pins—endosteal or endosseous or endodontic.
- Sub periosteal framework—subperiosteal implants.

Q. 201. What is endosteal implant?

Ans. Endosteal implant is a device placed into the alveolar and/or basal bone of the mandible or maxilla and transsecting only one cortical plate.

Q. 202. What is eposteal dental implant?

Ans. Eposteal dental implant is that implant which receives its primary bone support by means of resting on the alveolar bone.

Q. 203. What is transsosseous dental implant?

Ans. A dental implant that penetrates both cortical plates and passes through the full thickness of the alveolar bone is transosseous dental implant.

Q. 204. How do implants integrate with bone?

Ans. The implants may have the following:

- Fibrous integration
- Fibro-osseous integration
- Osseos integration.

Q. 205. Name the few implant systems.

Ans. There are numerous implant systems im the market from which the dentist can choose; for example, Nobel Biocare, Ankylos, Osstem, Myriad, Alpha Bio, Biohorizon.

Q. 206. What are the different materials used for implants?

Ans. Materials used for dental implants are:

- Metals
  - Stainless steel
  - Chrome-cobalt alloy

  - Titanium and its alloys
  - Surface coated titanium.
- Ceramics
  - Hydroxy appetite
  - Aluminum oxide
  - Bioglass
  - Tricalcium phosphate.
- Polymers and composites
  - Polymethyl methacrylate
  - Polytetra fluoro ethylene
  - Silicone rubber
  - Polysulfone
  - Polyethylene.
- Carbon
  - Polycrystalline carbon
  - Carbon silicone.

Q. 207. What are the advantages of implants supported prostheses?

Ans. Advantages of implant supported prostheses:

- Bone maintenance
- Restoring facial esthetics
- Improved occlusion
- Improved phonetics
- Improved masticatory performance and maintainence of muscles of mastication and facial expression
- Reduced size of prostheses
- Improved retention and stability of removable prostheses
- Increased survival time of prostheses
- Elimination of need to alter adjacent teeth
- More permanent replacement
- Improved pschyological health.

Q. 208. Define osseointegration.

Ans. Osseointegration or osseous-integration is the apparent direct attachment or connection of osseous tissue to an inert alloplastic material without intervening connective issue.

Q. 209. What are the factors responsible for successful osseointegration?

Ans.

- Implant material biocompatibility
- Loading conditions
- Implant design characteristic
- Surgical considerations
- Implant surface characteristic
- State of host bed.

Q. 210. What are the indications for dental implants?

Ans. Indications for implants are:

- Patient with partially or fully edentulous arches as long as they fulfill specific requirements for surgical and prosthetic rehabilitation
- Patients who are unable to wear removable dentures and have adequate bone for insertion of implants
- Poor oral muscular coordination
- Low tolerance of the mucosal tissue
- Unrealistic prosthodontic expectations.

Q. 211. What are contraindications for dental implants?

Ans. Contraindications for dental implants are:

- Uncontrolled diabetes, chronic, steroid therapy, high dose irradiation, alcohol, abuse and smoking.
- Pathologic conditions present in hard or soft tissue of either jaws

- Presence of untreated or unsuccessfully treated periodontal disease
- Any other systemic condition contraindicating surgery.

Q. 212. What are the steps involved in fabrication of an implant supported complete denture?

Ans. The steps involved are:

- Preliminary impression
- Final impression
- Interocclusal registration
- Trial denture
- Fabrication of the bar attachment
- Processing the overdenture
- Denture delivery.

Q. 213. What is a healing screw?

Ans. The healing screw or a cover screw is the component of an endosteal dental implant system used to seal usually on an interim basis, the implant body during the healing phase, after surgical placement.

The purpc se of healing screw is to maintain potency of the internal threaded section for subsequent attachment of abutment during second stage surgery.

Q. 214. Define implant abutment?

Ans. The portion of a dental implant that serves to support and/or retain any prosthesis is known as implant abutment.

Q. 215. What is transfer coping?

Ans. A transfer coping is used in traditional prosthesis to position a die in an impression, which is necessary to transfer the position and design of the implant or abutment to a master cast for prosthesis fabrication.

Q. 216. What is implant analog? Give other names for it.

Ans. An implant analog is used in the fabrication of the master cast to replicate the retentive portion of the implant body or abutment.

Implant analog is also known as abutment replica or implant body.

Q. 217. What is masticatory apparatus?

Ans. Masticatory apparatus is a system which consists of organs and structures primarily functioning in mastication. These include the teeth with their supporting structures, craniomandibular articulations, mandible positioning and accessory musculature, tongue, lips, cheeks, oral mucosa and the associate neurologic complex.

Q. 218. What is gnathology?

Ans. Gnathology is a science which deals with the masticatory apparatus as a whole including morphology, anatomy, histology, physiology, pathology and therapeutics.

Q. 219. What is denture stomatitis and how will you treat it?

Ans. Denture stomatitis, a chronic inflammation can be the following types:

- Type I - A localized inflammation
- Type II - A diffuse erythema involving the entire denture covered mucosa
- Type III- A granular type involving the central part of the hard palate and the alveolar ridge.

Treatment of denture stomatitis requires:

1. Removal of the cause—Discontinue dentures
2. Good oral and dental hygiene maintenance

3. Rest to tissues by removal of dentures or by use of tissues conditions along with occlusal adjustment
4. Antifungal therapy—Therapeutic dose of one nystatin tablets 3 times a day for 10-14 days
5. Mouthwash—Chlorhexidine.

Q. 220. What is denture sore mouth or burning mouth syndrome?

Ans. It is a vague burning sensation in one or several oral structures in contact with the dentures. It may be due to following factors:

- Local factors
  - Infection
  - Allergy
  - Mechanical irritation
  - Parafunctional habits.
- Systemic factors
  - Vitamin deficiency
  - Menopause
  - Diabetes
  - Xerostomia.
- Psychogenic factors
  - Depression
  - Anxiety.

Q. 221. What is denture granuloma?

Ans. Denture granuloma is a granular tumor or growth usually of lymphoid and epithelioid cells occurs due to denture trauma.

Q. 222. When should be the first recall for a complete denture patient?

Ans. The first recall for a complete denture patient should ideally be after 24 hours.

Q. 223. What are the causes of midline fracture of upper complete denture?

Ans. The midline fracture of upper complete denture may be caused by:

- Median tori
- Prominent mid palatal raphe
- Buccal placement of posterior teeth with heavy occlusion
- High labial frenal attachment close to the crest of the ridge.

Q. 224. What is the cause of pain while swallowing in complete denture patients?

Ans. Reason for pain while swallowing is due to the over extension of the lingual flange in the retromylohyoid area.

Q. 225. What is geriatric dentistry?

Ans. Geriatric dentistry is the branch of dental care involving problems peculiar to advanced age and aging.

Q. 226. Enumerate unconventional dentures.

Ans. Unconventional dentures are:

- Overdenture
- Immediate denture
- Implant denture
- Obturator with complete or partial denture.

Q. 227. What is residual ridge resorption?

Ans. Residual ridge resorption is a term used for the diminishing quantity and quality of residual ridge after teeth are extracted. It is referred as R.R.R. by D. A. Atwood.

Q. 228. Which are the different materials used for repair of complete denture? Which one is most preferred?

Ans. The materials used for repair of complete denture are:

- Self cure acrylic resin
- Heat cure acrylic resin
- Light cured resin repairs.

Self cure or light cured resins is the preferred material as it has simple procedure, avoids warpage of denture and saves time.

Q. 229. Name different medicaments used for complete denture patient?

Ans.

- Prior to commencing the complete denture treatment, the medicaments used are:
  - Gums paints.
- While treating the patient for complete dentures:
  - Gum paints
  - Oral mouth wash.
- After completion of the complete denture treatment:
  - Gum paints
  - Topical Anesthetic
  - Analgesic:
    - When painful ulcers occurs due to trauma from dentures
    - When gagging reflex is exaggerated local anesthetic application on soft palate reduces gagging.
  - Artificial saliva in patients with xerostomia
  - Antifungal treatment in cases with candidiasis.

CHAPTER

3

Removable Partial Dentures

Q. 1. What is a removable partial denture?

Ans. According to Glossary of Prosthodontic terms, any dental prosthesis that replaces some teeth in a partially dentate arch. It can be removed from the mouth and replaced at will.

Q. 2. What is a removable bridge?

Ans. It is a single tooth posterior removable partial denture with clasps on either sides, taking retention and support from the abutment teeth adjacent to the edentulous area.

Q. 3. What is an acrylic partial denture?

Ans. An artificial substitute for a few missing natural teeth and adjacent tissues made of acrylic resin, and is only tissue bound is known as acrylic partial denture. It is an interim denture.

Q. 4. What is the difference between acrylic and planned cast partial denture?

Ans. The difference between acrylic and planned cast partial denture is that acrylic cast partial denture is a soft tissue supported removable partial denture with wrought wire clasps to retain prosthesis. Whereas planned cast partial denture is a tooth or tooth-tissue supported RPD with a cast framework, which takes support and retention from the abutment teeth and soft tissues depending on the edentulous span.

Q. 5. What is an abutment?

Ans. An abutment is a tooth, a portion of a tooth or that portion of a dental implant that serves to support and/or retain a prosthesis.

Q. 6. What is an interim denture?

Ans. An interim denture is a fixed or removable prosthesis designed to enhance esthetics, stabilization and function for a limited period of time, after which it is to be replaced by a definitive prosthesis.

Q. 7. What is a transitional denture?

Ans. A dental prosthesis to be used for a short time for reasons of esthetics, mastication, occlusal support or convenience or for conditioning the patient to accept an artificial substitute for missing natural teeth until a more definite prosthetic dental treatment can be provided.

Q. 8. What is a treatment denture?

Ans. A treatment denture is a dental prosthesis used for the purpose of treating or conditioning the tissues that are called on to support and retain it.

Q. 9. What are the steps in fabrication of removable partial dentures?

Ans. The various steps in fabrication of removable partial dentures are as follows:

- Examination, diagnosis and treatment planning
  - Impressions for diagnostic cast
  - Diagnostic surveying.
- Treatment planning
- Mouth preparations
- Impressions for master cast
- Surveying of master cast—Definitive surveying
- Final treatment plan
- Block out of master cast
- Duplication of master cast
- Refractory cast
- Wax pattern on refractory cast
- Spruing, investing and casting
- Deinvesting and finishing of casting
- Fitting on master cast
- Fabrication of trays, if functional impression required
- Functional impression
- Modification of master cast to get altered cast
- Preparation of temporary bases for jaw relation
- Jaw relation
- Arrangement of teeth
- Try-in
- Processing of denture
- Denture delivery (relining for functional impression, if required)
- Follow-up.

Q. 10. What are the materials used for fabrication of removable partial dentures?

Ans. Materials for removable partial dentures are:

- Nonmetallic
  - Acrylic resins
  - Vinyl resins—flexible resins

- Metallic
  - Precious—IV gold alloys
  - Base metal alloys, chrome cobalt alloys
  - Titanium.

Q. 11. What is the purpose of classification in partially edentulous conditions?

Ans. The purposes of classification are:

- To allow visualization of the type of partially edentulous arch being considered
- To permit differentiation between tooth-supported and tooth-tissue supported partial dentures
- To serve as a guide to the type of design to be used
- To universally accept and discuss the condition.

Q. 12. What is Kennedy's classification for partially edentulous areas?

Ans. Kennedy's classification for partially edentulous areas are as follows:

- It contains four classes with certain modifications:
  - **Class I:** Bilateral edentulous areas located posterior to the remaining natural teeth
  - **Class II:** Unilateral edentulous area located posterior to the remaining natural teeth
  - **Class III:** Unilateral edentulous area with natural teeth both anterior and posterior to it
  - **Class IV:** A single, but bilateral (crossing the midline), edentulous area located anterior to the remaining natural teeth.
- Dr OC Applegate (1960) further added various modifications in this classification:
  - **Class V:** An edentulous area bounded anteriorly and posteriorly by natural teeth but in which the anterior abutment (lateral incisor) is not suitable for support.

- **Class VI:** Is an edentulous situation in which the teeth adjacent to the space are capable of the required prosthesis; it would occur most frequently in a young adult for whom a fixed partial denture is indicated but possible damage to the dental pulp might occur, if crown preparation were attempted.

Q. 13. What are the Applegate's rules to Kennedy's classification?

Ans.
- Classification should follow rather than precede extractions that might alter the original classification
- If the third molar is missing and not to be replaced it is not considered in the classification
- If the third molar is present and is to be used as an abutment, it is considered in the classification.
- If a second molar is missing and is not to be replaced (i.e. the opposing second molar is also missing and is not to be replaced); it is not used in the classification
- The most posterior edentulous area or areas always determine the classification
- Edentulous areas other than those determining the classification are referred to as modification spaces and are designated by their numbers
- The extent of the modification is not considered, only the number of additional edentulous areas
- There can be no modification areas in class IV arches. Any edentulous area lying posterior to the single bilateral area determines the classification.

Q. 14. What is a distal extension base partial denture?

Ans. Distal extension base partial denture is a removable partial denture that is supported and retained by natural teeth only at one end of the denture base segment and in which a portion of the functional load is carried by the residual ridge.

Q. 15. Differentiate Kennedy's classification I and II?

Ans. In class I, there is bilateral edentulous areas located posterior to the remaining natural teeth while in class II, there is unilateral edentulous area.

Q. 16. What is the classification, if only upper left central incisor in missing or upper left central incisor is present?

Ans. The classification if only upper left central incisor is missing would be class VI. If only upper left central incisor is present—class I.

Q. 17. Why Kennedy's class IV does not have any modification areas?

Ans. Kennedy's class IV does not have any modification area as the Applegate's rule 5 states that the most posterior edentulous areas should be considered first for determining the classification.

Q. 18. What is a modification area?

Ans. Edentulous areas other than those determining the classification are referred as modification areas. They are designated by the number of edentulous areas and not by the number of teeth missing.

Q. 19. Mention two Applegate's rules which govern Kennedy's classification.

Ans. Two of Applegate's rule which govern Kennedy's classification are:

Rule 1: Classification should follow rather than precede extractions that might alter the original classification.

Rule 2: If 3rd molar is missing and not to be replaced, it is not considered in the classification.

Q. 20. Name different partial denture components.

Ans. The different partial denture components are as follows:

- Major connectors
- Minor connectors
- Direct retainers
- Indirect retainers
- Denture bases
- Artificial teeth
- Stress breaker (optional).

Q. 21. What is a major connector?

Ans. A major connector is that part of a removable partial denture that connects the parts of the prosthesis located on one side of the arch with those on the opposite side.

Q. 22. Why major connector must be rigid?

Ans. Rigidity allows stresses that are applied to any portion of the partial denture to be effectively distributed over the entire supporting area including the abutment teeth, other teeth included in the design in partial denture, underlying bone and soft issue.

Q. 23. What are the different types of maxillary major connectors?

Ans. The different types of maxillary major connectors are:

- Single posterior palatal bar
- Palatal strap
- Anteroposterior or double palatal bar
- Horse shoe or U-shaped connector
- Closed horseshoe
- Complete palate.

Q. 24. What are the various mandibular major connectors?

Ans. The various mandibular major connectors are:

- Lingual bar
- Lingual plate or linguo plate
- Continuous bar retainer
- Cut back lingual plate
- Sub lingual bar
- Labial bar.

Q. 25. What should be the ideal location for palatal bar or lingual bar and why?

Ans. The ideal location for a palatal bar is center of the dental arch and no further anterior than the second premolar position. Because any further anterior placement will cause severe interference with action of the tongue.

The ideal location of lingual bar is as inferior as the patient can tolerate not only to permit more freedom of movement for the tongue, but also to permit more space between the marginal gingival and the superior border of the bar to avoid adverse soft tissue response like hypertrophy or hyperplasia. It should be 3 mm lower than the free gingival margin.

Q. 26. What are the indications for a linguoplate?

Ans. The indications for a linguoplate are:

- When the lingual frenum is high or the space available for a lingual bar is limited
- In class I situation in which residual ridges have undergone excessive vertical resorption.
- For stabilizing periodontally weakened teeth
- When further replacement of one or more teeth is required
- When there is need for indirect retention.

Q. 27. What are the indications of labial bar major connector?

Ans. It is indicated in case of lingually tilted anterior and posterior teeth (non-correctable) and in presence of large lingual tori.

Q. 28. Define minor connectors.

Ans. Minor connectors are the connecting link between the major connector or base of a removable partial denture and the other units of the prosthesis, such as the clasp assembly, indirect retainers, occlusal rests or cingulum rest.

Q. 29. What are the functions of minor connectors?

Ans. The functions of minor connectors are:

- To join denture parts
- To transfer functional stress to the abutment teeth
- To transfer the effect of the retainers, rests and stabilizing components to the rest of the denture
- It attaches the denture base to the teeth.

Q. 30. What are the types of minor connectors?

Ans. The various types of minor connectors are:

- Minor connectors that join clasp assembly to major connector
- Minor connectors that join indirect retainers or auxiliary rests to major connector
- Minor connectors that join the denture base with the major connector
- Minor connectors that serve as approach arm for vertical projection or bar type clasp.

Q. 31. What is rest in removable partial denture?

Ans. The components of a removable partial denture that serve primarily to transfer forces from the prosthesis down the long axis of the abutment teeth are called rests.

It is that component of a removable partial denture that acquires support from the occlusal rest seat.

Q. 32. Name the different types of rest. Why lingual rest is preferable to incisal rest?

Ans. The different types of rest are:

- Occlusal rest
  - Conventional
  - Extended
  - Overlay.
- Cingulum rest
- Incisal rest.

Cingulum rest is preferable to incisal rest because of the following reasons:

- Cingulum rest is nearer to the center of rotation of the supporting tooth, as it does not tend to tip the tooth
- More esthetically acceptable
- Resultant forces on partial denture passing through a lingual rest are of less mangnitude than taking place against an incisal rest.

Q. 33. What are auxillary occlusal rests?

Ans. Auxillary occlusal rests means additional rests. These are not a part of the direct retainers, but rests given on other occlusal surfaces, for support or indirect retention.

Q. 34. What will be the consequences, if angle between occlusal rest and minor connector is more than 90 degrees?

Ans. An angle greater than 90 degrees will not transmit the forces vertically, but will create an inclined plane effect. This inclined plane could produce slippage of the prosthesis away from the abutment tooth, which would place unnecessary strain on other supporting teeth. The inclined plane can also cause orthodontic movement of abutment tooth with concurrent pain and bone loss.

Q. 35. Explain internal rest.

Ans. A partial denture that is totally tooth supported by means of cast retainers on all abutment teeth may use internal occlusal rests for both occlusal support and horizontal stabilization. It is a rest housed within the coronal structure of the tooth with parallel walls and a definite seat.

Q. 36. What is a direct retainer?

Ans. Direct retainer is that component of a removable partial denture used to retain and prevent dislodgement, consisting of a clasp assembly or precision attachment.

Q. 37. Classify direct retainers.

Ans. Direct retainers are classified as:

- Intracoronal direct retainer
  - Internal attachment
  - External attachment
  - Stud attachment
  - Bar attachment
  - Special attachment.
- Extracoronal direct retainers
  - Manufactured retainers (Dalbo)
  - Custom-made retainers
    - Occlusally approaching (Aker's or circumference)

    ¤ Gingivally approaching (bar or roach).
  - Metal-cast metal
    ¤ Wrought metal.

Q. 38. What is an intracoronal direct retainer?

Ans. An intracoronal direct retainer is that part of removable partial denture, which engages vertical walls built into the crown of the abutment tooth to create frictional resistance to removal.

Q. 39. What are the limitations to the use of intracoronal direct retainers?

Ans. The limitation to the use of intracoronal direct retainers are:

- They require prepared abutments and castings
- They require complicated clinical and laboratory procedures
- They eventually wear, with resulting loss of frictional resistance to denture removal
- They are difficult to repair and replace
- They are least effective on short teeth
- They are difficult to place completely within the circumference of an abutment tooth.

Q. 40. What are the advantages and disadvantages of suprabulge or cast circumferential or Akers clasp?

Ans. Advantages

- Simplicity of design
- Easy construction
- Provides excellent support, bracing and retentive properties
- Close adaptation to tooth surface so, no food entrapment.

Disadvantages

- Large amount of tooth covered, so underlying enamel is prone to decalcification.
- The display of metal
- Alters the gross morphology of the clinical crown interfering with food flow pattern compromising periodontal health
- Difficulty in adjusting.

Q. 41. What are the different types of cast circumferential clasps?

Ans.

- Simple circlet clasp
- Reverse circlet design
- Multiple circlet clasp
- Embrasure clasp
- Ring clasp
- C-clasp (reverse action, hairpin or fishhook clasp)
- Onlay clasp design
- Half-and-half clasp
- Extended arm clasp.

Q. 42. What is angle of cervical convergence?

Ans. Angle of cervical convergence is the angle formed by any surface of the tooth below the survey line or the height of contour with the selected path of insertion of a prosthesis.

Q. 43. What are the components of an extracoronal direct retainer?

Ans. The components of an extracoronal direct retainer are:

- Retentive arm

- Stabilizing arm/reciprocal arm
- Occlusal rest
- Minor connector.

Q. 44. What are the principles of designing a clasp?

Ans. The principles of designing a clasp are:

- Retention
- Stability
- Reciprocation
- Support
- Encirclement more than 180°
- Passive
- Esthetics.

Q. 45. What are the factors on which flexibility of retentive clasp arm depend on?

Ans. Flexibility of retentive clasp arm depends on:

- Length of clasp (directly proportional)
- Diameter of clasp arm (inversely proportional)
- Taper
- Cross-sectional form—round or half round
- Material
  - Gold
  - Chrome cobalt
  - Titanium
  - Wrought or cast.

Q. 46. Where is the retentive tip placed?

Ans. It is placed in the gingival 1/3rd below the height of contour.

Q. 47. What are the functions of reciprocal tip?

Ans. The functions of reciprocal arm are:

- Reciprocation against the action of the retentive arm
- Stabilization against horizontal movement.

Q. 48. Where should the reciprocal arm be located?

Ans. Reciprocal arm should be located above the height of contour on the opposite side of retentive arm at the middle and gingival third of the tooth.

Q. 49. What are the indications for the use of a ring clasp?

Ans. The indications for a ring clasp are:

- An isolated mesially titled molar
- When proximal undercut cannot be approached by other means.

Q. 50. Why embrasure clasp must have double occusal rest?

Ans. Embrasure clasp must have double occlusal rest in order to:

- Avoid interproximal wedging by the prosthesis which could cause separation of the abutment teeth and result in food impaction and clasp displacement
- Provide support and also serve to shunt food away from contact area.

Q. 51. What is a roach clasp?

Ans. Roach clasp is a vertical projection or bar clasp which approaches the undercut retentive area on tooth from a gingival direction resulting in "push" type of retention.

Q. 52. What are the advantages and disadvantages of infrabulge clasp?

Ans. Advantages

- Minimal tooth contact and minimal distortion of normal tooth contours
- Improved esthetics

- Increased retention because of tripping action Decreased torquing forces applied to terminal abutments in extension removable partial dentures
- Improved adjustability because the location of the bend is less critical than for circumferential clasps.

Disadvantages

- They cannot be used in the presence of soft tissue undercuts, a shallow vestibule or high frenal attachments
- Bracing action provided by bar clasps is considerably less than that provided by cast circumferential clasps
- The bar clasp will not totally disengage in certain distal extension cases (where the undercut is located on the distofacial surface of the terminal abutment)
- Appearance may be adversely affected, if the smile line is high enough to expose the approach arm as it crosses the gingiva
- They may not be retentive unless rigid elements determine a specific path of insertion/dislodgment.

Q. 53. What are the types of infrabulge clasps?

Ans.
- T-clasp
- Modified T–clasp
- Y-clasp
- I clasp.

Q. 54. What are the advantages of a combination clasp?

Ans. It is introduced by Dr OC Applegate in 1965. The advantages of a combination clasp lie in the flexibility, adjustability and appearance of wrought wire retentive arm.

The advantages are:

- Due to flexibility of wrought wire it acts as a stress equalizer, preventing undesirable forces created by the lever action of the retentive clasp tip from lifting or torquing the abutment tooth as downward forces occur on denture base
- Can be placed in a greater or deeper undercut due to its flexibility.
- More esthetically pleasing in appearance
- Can be adjusted in all planes
- Round wire makes only line contact with the surface of abutment tooth rather than the area contact of a cast clasp indicated in patients with high decay-missing-filled (DMF) index
- Less fatigue failures.

Q. 55. What is RPI clasp system?

Ans. RPI clasp system stands for R-Rest; P-Proximal plate and I-I bar. This system consists of a mesiooclusal rest with minor connector placed in mesiolingual embrasure but not contacting adjacent tooth. Proximal plate on the distal surface I bar placed on the buccal surface (mesial undercut or maximum of tooth bulk). It is a concept introduced by AJ Krol in 1973.

Q. 56. What are the contraindications for the use of RPI clasp?

Ans. The contraindication for use of RPI clasp are:

- Buccal or lingual tilts of abutment teeth
- Severe tissue undercut
- Shallow buccal vestibule
- Desirable undercut is located on distal surface of tooth.

Q. 57. What is a RPA clasp system?

Ans. RPA is modification of RPI retainer, devised by Krol in 1980. I bar was replaced with an Aker's clasp in patients with soft tissue undercuts and high frenal attachments.

Q. 58. What is a fulcrum line in removable partial dentures?

Ans. According to Glossary Prosthodontics terms, an imaginary line, connecting occlusal rests, around which a removable partial denture tends to rotate under masticatory forces. The determinants for the fulcrum line are usually the cross arch occlusal rests located adjacent to the tissue borne components.

Q. 59. What is an indirect retainer?

Ans. According to Glossary Prosthodontics terms, indirect retainer is that component of a removable partial denture that assists the direct retainer(s) in preventing displacement of the distal extension denture base by functioning through lever action on the opposite side of fulcrum line when denture base moves away from tissues in pure rotation around the fulcrum line.

Q. 60. What are the forms of indirect retainers?

Ans. The forms of indirect retainers are:

- Auxillary occlusal rests
- Canine extension from occlusal rest
- Canine rest
- Continuous bar retainer and linguoplates
- Modification areas
- Rugae support
- Direct indirect retention
- Major connector.

Q. 61. Define a denture base.

Ans. Denture base is the part of a denture that rests on the foundation tissues and to which teeth are attached.

Q. 62. What decides the need for relining of partial denture base?

Ans.
- Visual references to loss of supporting tissue established due to resportion of residual ridge. Evaluated by space under denture base by thin mix of alginate
- When pressure is applied on the distal extension base partial dentures, the indirect retainer lifts up indicating loss of tissue support.

Q. 63. Why should distal extension bases be made in acrylic resin?

Ans. Distal extension bases should be made in acrylic resin because:
- It can be easily relined or rebased to reestablish tissue support
- It can be modified at the borders, if adjustment is required.

Q. 64. What is a stress breaker?

Ans. According to Glossary, stress breaker is a device or system that relieves specific dental structures of part or all of the occlusal forces and redirects those forces to other bearing structures or regions.

Q. 65. What are the aims of stress breaking?

Ans. Various aims of stress breaking are as follows:
- To direct occlusal forces in the long axis of the abutment teeth
- To prevent harmful loads being applied to the remaining natural teeth

- To share load as evenly as possible between the natural teeth and saddle areas according to the ability of these different tissues to accept the loads
- To ensure that part of the load applied to the saddle area is distributed as evenly as possible over the whole mucosal surface
- To provide greater comfort to the patient.

Q. 66. What are the main biological considerations while designing the partial denture?

Ans. While designing partial dentures, the residual ridge and abutment teeth are the factors to be considered.

Q. 67. What are the points of differences between tooth supported and tooth-tissue supported partial denture?

Ans. Differences between tooth supported and tooth-tissue supported partial denture are as follows:

Tooth supported partial denture	*Tooth-tissue supported partial denture*
1. Short span class III derives support from abutment teeth	1. Class I and class II derives support from abutment teeth partially and partially from tissues
2. Functional impression not required	2. Functional impression required
3. Indirect retention is not required	3. Indirect retention is required
4. Metallic or resin base is indicated	4. Resin denture base is indicated for feasibility of relining

Q. 68. What are the different fulcrum lines in removable partial dentures?

Ans. The different fulcrum line are:

- One fulcrum line is on horizontal plane that extends through the two principal abutments one on each side of dental arch
- Second fulcrum is on the sagittal plane and extends through the occlusal rest on the terminal abutment and along the crest of residual ridge on one side of the arch
- Third fulcrum, a vertical line is located in the vicinity of the midline just lingual to the anterior teeth.

Q. 69. What are the movements of removable partial denture?

Ans. The movements of removable partial denture are:

- Towards or away from the supporting ridge (rotational movement of denture in sagittal plane)
- Side to side movements over the crest ridge or rocking (rotational movement in vertical plane)
- Rotational movement of denture in horizontal plane or flat circular movements of denture.

Q. 70. What is a dental surveyor?

Ans. Dental surveyor is a paralleling instrument used in construction of prosthesis to locate and delineate the contours and relative positions of abutment teeth and associated structures.

Q. 71. What is surveying?

Ans. An analysis and comparison of the prominence of intraoral contours associated with the fabrication of a prosthesis.

Q. 72. What is path of insertion? Which factors help in deciding path of insertion?

Ans. **According to Glossary:** The specific direction in which a prosthesis is placed on the abutment teeth.

According to Stewart: The tilt of the cast on the surveyor is contemplated to determined at what angle the partial denture will seat over the remaining teeth and any other obstructions that may be present.

This path that the prosthesis follows, as it goes into place is referred to as the path of insertion of the denture.

The factors which help in deciding path of insertion are:

- Retentive undercuts
- Guiding planes
- Interferences
- Esthetics.

Q. 73. What are guiding planes?

Ans. **According to Glossary,** guiding planes are vertically parallel surfaces of abutment teeth oriented so as to contribute to the direction of the path of placement and removal of a removable partial denture.

Q. 74. What is tripoding or tripod marking?

Ans. The marks or lines drawn on a cast in a single plane perpendicular to the survey rod to assist with repositioning the cast on a dental surveyor in a previously defined orientation **is known as tripoding**.

Q. 75. What is height of contour?

Ans. Height of contour is a line encircling a tooth and designating its greatest circumferences at a selected axial position determined by a dental surveyor.

Q. 76. What is diagnostic cast?

Ans. **According to Glossary,** diagnostic cast is a life-size reproduction of a part or parts of the oral cavity and/

or facial structures for the purpose of study and treatment planning.

Q. 77. What are the index areas (radiographic)?

Ans. Index areas are those areas of alveolar support that disclose the reaction of bone to additional stress.

Q. 78. What is mouth preparation?

Ans. The preparations done in the mouth either surgical or nonsurgical to receive the designed removable partial denture favorably is known as mouth preparation.

Q. 79. What are the abutment modifications required for a removable partial denture?

Ans. The required abutment modifications are as follows:

- Preparation of guide planes
- Recontouring buccal/lingual surface for repositioning height of contour
- Dimpling
- Rest seat preparation
- Tooth preparation for full crown, if indicated.

Q. 80. How the presence of tori will affect the partial denture design?

Ans. The presence of tori will cause:

- Additional stresses to supporting elements and compromised function
- Cause irritation and chronic ulceration of tissues covered
- It requires relief while designing
- If the tori is large, it should not be covered in the partial denture design.

Q. 81. What is the objective of periodontal therapy for partially edentulous patient?

Ans. The objective of periodontal therapy for partially edentulous patient is the return to health of the supporting structures of the teeth, creating an environment in which the periodontium may be maintained.

Q. 82. Why an abutment teeth should be prepared?

Ans. Abutment teeth should be prepared to provide support, stabilization, reciprocation and retention for the partial denture.

Q. 83. What is anatomic form and functional form of ridges?

Ans. The anatomic form of ridge is the surface contour of the ridge when it is not recorded under occlusal load and denotes the resting form of the ridge.

The form of residual ridge recorded under functional loading, whether by occlusal loading, finger loading, specially designed individual trays or consistency of recording medium is called functional form of ridge. It is the supporting state of the ridges.

Q. 84. What do you mean by tissue placement?

Ans. The change in the form and position of tissues as a result of pressure under physiological limits is known as tissue placement.

Q. 85. What is the most favorable path of insertion of a removable partial denture?

Ans. The most favorable path of insertion of a removable partial denture is one perpendicular to the occlusal plane.

Q. 86. What should be the size of artificial teeth used to replace the missing posterior teeth in removable partial denture?

Ans. The artificial teeth used to replace the missing posterior teeth in removable partial denture should be 2/3rd of the faciolingual width of the natural teeth and the cusp angles should be shallow.

Q. 87. What should be the shape of a lingual bar in cross section?

Ans. Lingual bar should be half pear-shaped with the thin portion facing the gingiva and thick portion towards, the sulcus.

Q. 88. What are the commonly used duplicating material?

Ans.
- Agar
- Silicone
- Alginate.

Q. 89. In which of the Kennedy's class, functional impression is required to be made?

Ans. Functional impressions are required to be made in Kennedy's class I and class II situations. In addition, when the tissues on the edentulous ridge are compressible and required to be recorded for maximum support.

Q. 90. What is the objectives of making a functional impression in distal extension base partial dentures?

Ans. The objective of functional impression technique is to provide maximum support for the removable partial denture base, thereby occlusal contact to distribute the occlusal load over both natural and artificial dentition and, at the same time, movement of the base is minimized, which would create leverage on abutment teeth.

Q. 91. What are the different methods for functional impression technique?

Ans. The different methods for functional impression technique are:

- Physiologic
  - Mclean's and Hindal's technique
  - Fluidwax technique—Altered cast technique
  - Functional relining—At denture delivery.
- Selective pressure technique—Altered cast technique.

Q. 92. How will you check the errors in occlusion after processing a removable partial denture?

Ans. The errors in occlusion after processing a removable partial denture can be checked only by patient remount.

Q. 93. What is swing lock removable partial denture?

Ans. In the swing lock removable partial denture, all or several of the remaining teeth are used to retain and stabilize the prosthesis against vertical displacement. Prosthesis consists of a hinged buccal or labial bar attached to a conventional major connector.

CHAPTER

4

Fixed Partial Dentures

Q. 1. Define a fixed partial denture?

Ans. A fixed partial denture is a restoration which replaces few of the natural teeth and which cannot be readily removed by the patient or dentist, it is permanently attached to the natural teeth or roots which furnish the primary support.

Q. 2. What are the different components of a fixed partial denture?

Ans. The different components of a fixed partial denture are:

- Retainers
- Pontic
- Connector.

Q. 3. Classify fixed partial denture?

Ans. Depending on the type of connectors:

- Fixed fixed partial denture
- Fixed movable partial denture
- Removable fixed partial denture.

- Depending on the type of materials used:
  - All metal crown
  - Metal ceramic crown
  - All ceramic crown
  - All acrylic crown
  - Ceramic veneer
  - Acrylic veneer.
- Depending on length of edentulous span:
  - Short span bridge
  - Long span bridges.
- Depending on duration of use:
  - Permanent fixed partial denture
  - Provisional fixed partial denture.

Q. 4. What is a retainer?

Ans. It is that component of a fixed partial denture which attaches the prosthesis to the abutments.

Q. 5. What is a pontic?

Ans. A pontic is defined as the suspended member of a fixed partial denture replacing, the lost natural tooth, restoring its function and usually occupying the space of the missing natural tooth.

Q. 6. What is a connector?

Ans. A connector is that part of a fixed partial denture that unite its component parts, i.e. the pontic and retainer.

Q. 7. Define an abutment.

Ans. An abutment is a tooth or root used for the support or attachment of a fixed partial denture or removable partial denture.

Q. 8. What is a pier abutment?

Ans. A pier abutment is a natural tooth or root without other natural teeth in proximal contact, which is used as an abutment in addition to two terminal abutment.

Q. 9. What is a bridge?

Ans. It may defined as a partial prosthesis rigidly cemented to one or more teeth and replacing one or more but not all natural teeth.

Q. 10. What are the different types of bridges?

Ans. The different types of bridges are:

- Fixed-fixed bridge
- Fixed movable bridge
- Modified fixed removable bridge —Andrew bridge
- Spring bridge
- Cantilever bridge
- Compound bridge
- Adhesive bridge.

Q. 11. What are the indications of a fixed partial denture?

Ans. Fixed partial dentures are indicated in the following situations:

- Short span edentulous arches
- Presence of sound tooth structure (crown or root) that can offer sufficient support adjacent to the edentulous space
- Preference for fixed restoration
- Physically handicapped patients who cannot maintain the removable prosthesis
- Patients suffering from epilepsy or other conditions whereby may have bouts of unconsciousness.
- Mentally compromised patients.

Q. 12. What are the contraindications of a fixed partial denture?

Ans. Fixed partial dentures are contraindicated in the following situations:

- Long span edentulous spaces
- Very young patients where pulp chamber is large
- Periodontally compromised abutments
- Large amount of bone loss
- Patients who cannot cooperate and spend time in a dental chair
- Older patients.

Q. 13. What is the importance of mounted diagnostic casts?

Ans. Mounted diagnostic casts serve the following purposes:

- To assess the dimensions of the edentulous space
- The height, rotations and inclination of abutments
- The number, size and position of wear facets can be seen
- Occlusion can be analysed.

Q. 14. What are the different types of connectors?

Ans. The different types of connectors are as follows:

- Rigid connectors
  - Cast
  - Soldered
- Non-rigid connectors
  - Tenon-mortise
  - Loop connectors
  - Split pontic
  - Cross pin and wing connectors
  - Dove-tail.

Q. 15. What are the indications and contraindications of rigid connectors?

Ans. Rigid connectors can be either cast as a single unit or joined by soldering. Soldering can be performed either before ceramic application (preceramic) or after ceramic application (postceramic).

Indications

- They are used to unite retainers and pontics in a fixed-fixed partial denture
- These connectors are used when the entire load on the pontic is to be transfered directly to the abutments.

Contraindications

- In cases where existing diastema is to be maintained
- In case of tilted abutments
- In abutments with differing long axis
- In long span bridges.

Q. 16. What are the indications to use non-rigid connectors?

Ans. There are several situations in which the use of non-rigid connectors is indicated either to relieve stress or to accommodate malaligned fixed partial denture abutments.

Q. 17. When would you indicate a cantilever bridge?

Ans. Cantilever bridge is indicated when there are:

- Missing maxillary lateral incisors
- Missing lower first premolar
- Missing second molar, when there in no distal abutment.

Q. 18. When would you indicate a fixed-fixed bridge?

Ans. Fixed-fixed bridge is indicated in:

1. In short span bridge situation
2. When splinting is required.

Q. 19. When would you indicate a fixed-movable bridge?

Ans. Fixed-movable bridge is indicated when one of the abutment is weak.

Q. 20. What are the requirements of an ideal abutment?

Ans. An ideal abutment should posses the following:

- Vital tooth
- Good bone support
- Proper arch form
- Proportional relationship between the crown and root is adequate.

Q. 21. Classify the retainers.

Ans. Retainers are classified as follows:

Extracoronal:

- Complete:
  - Anterior
  - Posterior.
- Partial:
  - Anterior—3/4
  - Posterior—4/5
    - ¤ 7/8
    - ¤ Mesial half: Mesial hood, Kennedy's Carmichael crown

Intracoronal:

- Pin ledge
- Onlays
- Inlays.

Radicular:

- Dowels-preformed
- Custom dowel with cores
  - Cast
  - Amalgam
  - Resin
  - Gold.
- Cast post and core.

Q. 22. Classify crowns.

Ans. Anterior crowns:

- Partial
  - Metal
  - Composite
  - Ceromer
  - Ceramic.
- Complete
  - Ceramic
  - Composite
  - Metal ceramic
  - Metal Composite
  - Ceromers.

Posterior crowns:

- Metal
- Composite
- Ceromer
- Ceramic
- Metal Ceramic.

Radicular crowns/dowel crowns.

Q. 23. What is a dowel crown?

Ans. Any one of the various types of artificial crowns or any combination, that is held in position by means of a dowel or post that extends into the root canal is a dowel crown.

Or

They are crowns with dowels which extend into the prepared root canal, used when it is impossible to restore the tooth by means of other restoration.

Q. 24. Classify dowel crown.

Ans. They can be classified according to:

- The type of dowel:
  - Wrought metal dowel

- Manufactured type (preformed)
- Cast metal dowel (cast core).

- The types of crown:
  - All metal with dowel
  - All porcelain with dowel.
    - ¤ Detached—Davis
    - ¤ Attached—Logan.
  - Combination of metal and porcelain with dowel
    - ¤ Richmond crown.
  - Combination of metal and plastic with dowel
  - All plastic with dowel.

Q. 25. What are the different core materials?

Ans. The different core materials are:

- Composite resin
- Amalgam
- Glass ionomer/reinforced glass ionomer
- Custom made cast core with post.

Q. 26. Classify post and core system.

Ans. Post/dowel system is classified into:

- Prefabricated posts
  - According to retention
    - ¤ Active
    - ¤ Passive.
  - According to shape
    - ¤ Tapered
    - ¤ Parallel.
  - According to material used
    - ¤ Metallic

- Platinum
- Gold
- Palladium
- Nickel-chromium

- Titanium.
    - ¤ Nonmetallic
- Ceramic
- Carbon-fiber post
- Fiber reinforced resin post.
- Cast post and core or custom made post and core
    - Direct
    - Indirect.

Q. 27. What are the factors that influence the design of a fixed prosthesis?

Ans. The following factors influence the design of a fixed prosthesis:

- Crown length
- Crown form
- Degree of mutilation
- Root length and form
- Crown Root ratio
- Ante's Law
- Periodontal health
- Span length
- Axial alignment
- Ach form
- Pulped health
- Alveolar bone loss
- Age of the patient
- Phonetics
- Esthetics
- Psychological factor.

Q. 28. What is Ante's Law?

Ans. Ante's law states that the total pericemental area of the abutment teeth should be equal or more than that of the teeth being replaced with pontics.

Q. 29. What are the biological principles of tooth preparation?

Ans. The biological principles of tooth preparation are:

- Conservation of tooth structure
- Avoidance of overheating—use of water coolent and intermittent preparations
- Avoidance of overcontouring
- Supragingival margin placement
- Protection against tooth fracture
- Protection of adjacent teeth.

Q. 30. What is biological width?

Ans. Biological width is the combined width of connective tissue and epithelial attachments superior to the crestal bone.

Q. 31. What is the significance of biological width?

Ans. Biological width should be maintained, violation of biological width causes loss of bone and connective tissue attachment, which leads to the migration of the epithelial attachment.

Q. 32. During which clinical situations, biological width is a concerned?

Ans. Biological width is of huge concern during:

- Tooth preparation procedures
- Restorative procedures
- Periodontal surgical procedure like crown lengthening.

Q. 33. What are the mechanical principles in tooth preparation?

Ans. The mechanical principles of tooth preparation are:

- Retention form to achieve retention in the restoration

- Resistance form to achieve resistance in the restoration
- Preventing deformation of restoration.

Q. 34. What are the esthetic principles in tooth preparation?

Ans. The esthetics principles in tooth preparation are:

- Adequate preparation to achieve esthetics
- Minimum display of metal
- Maximum thickness of porcelain
- Porcelain occlusal surfaces
- Subgingival margins.

Q. 35. What are the indications for a jacket crown?

Ans. Indications for a jacket crown are:

- Discolored teeth
- Incisal 1/3 fractured
- Large proximal cavities
- Malformed teeth
- When teeth are rotated and orthodontic treatment is not feasible
- Hypoplastic enamel—Mottled teeth.

Q. 36. How will you achieve retention in jacket crown preparation?

Ans. Retention is achieved by:

- Maintaining the length of the tooth
- Maintaining proximal surfaces parallel to each other
- Maintaining the labial and the cingulum portion parallel.

Q. 37. What are the two functions of a shoulder?

Ans. The two functions are:

- Bulk and strength of the crown
- Resistance to apical displacement.

Q. 38. Which type of a retainer (complete or partial) would you indicate in a patient with a high decayed missing filled (DMF) index?

Ans. In a patient with a high DMF index, a complete crown should be indicated.

Q. 39. What is the direction and placement of the axioproximal grooves in an anterior partial veneer crown?

Ans. They are placed:

- Parallel to the incisal 2/3rd of the labial surface
- Parallel to each other
- Taper from incisal to cervical end
- No definite seat at the gingival end.

Q. 40. What burs are used to prepare the incisal groove and proximal groove for anterior 3/4th partial veneer crown?

Ans.
- Incisal groove is prepared by using an inverted cone stone by placing the base of the inverted cone stone lingually and the sides facing liability
- Proximal grooves are prepared by using 700 cross cut fissure bur. Use low speed for their preparation.

Q. 41. What is the direction and placement of the axioproximal groove in the posterior 3/4th partial veneer crown?

Ans.
- The grooves are placed parallel to the long axis of the tooth
- They are at the junction of the buccal 1/3rd and lingual 2/3rd of the proximal surface
- They are parallel to each other
- They have a definite seat at the cervical end.

Q. 42. How much of the dowel pin should extend into the root canal?

Ans. The dowel pin should extend at least 2/3rd of the length of the root canal.

Or

It should extend at least equal to the length of the clinical crown which is to be replaced.

Q. 43. How would you open the root canal to receive a dowel?

Ans. The root canal is open:

- By a root canal instrument or pezo reamer
- By a ½ round bur.

Q. 44. What are the values of radiographs in fixed restoration?

Ans. Radiographs would help us to visualize the following:

- Size, shape and length of the root
- Size and position of the pulp
- Condition of the supporting tissues
- Condition of the supporting bone
- Crown to root ratio
- Angulation of the teeth
- Presence of pathology
- Trabecular bone pattern
- Undiscovered caries
- Assessment of previous filling.

Q. 45. What are the different types of finishing lines and give their indication?

Ans. The finishing lines can be:

- Subgingival
- Supragingival
- Equigingival.

They can be of the following types:

- Shoulder—All ceramic crown
- Chamfer/modified Chamfer—metal ceramic restoration
- Knife edge metal restoration
- Shoulder less or feather edge
- Modified shoulder with level—metal ceramic restoration
- Only Chamfer—metal restoration.

Q. 46. When would you indicate a subgingival finishing line?

Ans. A subgingival finish line is indicated in the following:

- For esthetics
- For retention in short crowns
- Extension for prevention of dental caries
- Large proximal contact
- Root sensitivity.

Q. 47. What is gingival retraction?

Ans. The deflection of the marginal gingival away from a tooth.

Q. 48. When is gingival retraction done?

Ans. Gingival retraction can be done:

- While preparation of the gingival finishing line
- Prior to making impression
- At cementation of a restoration.

Q. 49. What are the different types of gingival retraction methods?

Ans. They are:

- Mechanical—cords
  - Copper bands

  - Crowns
  - Rubber dam.
- Mechanico chemical—cords (knitted)
  - Braided
  - Cords with chemical aluminum
- Chemical
- Surgical
  - Scalpel
  - Rotary curretage—Gingettage
  - Electrosurgery
  - Laser.

Q. 50. What is a provisional restoration?

Ans. A fixed or removable prosthesis, designed to enhance esthetics stabilization and/or function for a limited period of time, after which it is to be replaced by a definitive prosthesis. Often such prostheses are used to assist in determination of the therapeutic effectiveness of a specific treatment plan or the form and function of the planned definitive prosthesis.

Q. 51. What are the different types of the provisional restoration?

Ans. Types of provisional restoration are as follows:

- Cast metal crowns
- Aluminum shell crown
- Cellulose acetate crown matrix
- Polycarbonate crown forms
- Heat cured acrylic resin treatment restoration
- Self cured acrylic resin treatment restoration
- Template matrix
- Post crown technique

- Preformed metal crown
- Composite crowns.

Q. 52. What are the provisional restorations for anterior teeth?

Ans. In the anterior region, esthetics is of prime importance. Cellulose acetate crown matrix or polycarbonate crown form, acrylic resin or composite resin crowns can be used as provisional for anterior teeth restoration.

Q. 53. What are the temporary cements?

Ans. Temporary cements used for cementation of provisional restorations are:

- Zinc oxide eugenol cement is used with metal restoration
- Noneugenol cement is used with resin restoration.

Q. 54. What are the cements used for definitive cementation?

Ans. The cements used for definitive cementation are:

- Glass ionomer cements
- Resin-modified glass ionomer cements
- Resin-luting
  - Light cured
  - Chemically cured
  - Dual cured.
- Zinc phosphate cement
- Zinc polycarboxylate cement.

Q. 55. What is die?

Ans. A die is a positive replica of a single tooth which has been prepared from a single tooth impression or a full arch impression.

Q. 56. What are the requirements of an ideal die material?

Ans. The following are the requirements of small an ideal die material:

- High strength
- Good resistance
- Should reproduce fine details
- Dimensionally stable
- Good color contrast
- Simple technique.

Q. 57. Enumerate the various die systems.

Ans. The various removable die systems are:

- Working cast with separate die system
- Working cast with removable die system
    - Dowel pin system
        - ¤ Straight pin (single)
    - Sleeve—plastic and metal
    - Without sleeve.
        - ¤ Straight (twin)
    - Sleeve—plastic and metal
    - Without sleeve.
        - ¤ Cured pin.
    - Di-lok tray system
    - Pindex system.
- Accutrac system
    - For ceramic laminate preparation.

Q. 58. What is a die-spacer?

Ans. Die spacer is a paint like material applied on the surface of a die prior to preparing the wax pattern. This provides for space in the final restoration for cement.

Q. 59. Classify die materials.

Ans. Die materials can be classified as:

Metallic	*Non- metallic*
Amalgam	Gypsum—Types IV and V
Electroform -Copper electroform -Silver electroform	Resin—epoxy resin
	Cement silico phosphate
	Flexible die material

Q. 60. What are the different elastomeric impression materials?

Ans. The elastomeric impression materials are classified as:

- According to chemistry
  - Polysulfide
  - Addition condensation silicone
  - Polyether
  - Light cured elastomer.
- According to viscosity
  - Putty
  - Heavy body
  - Medium body
  - Monophase
  - Light body
  - Ultralight body.

Q. 61. What are the techniques for impression making in fixed partial dentures?

Ans. Impression techniques can be classified based on the type of impression tray:

- Stock tray/putty wash impression
  - Double mix
  - Single mix.
- Custom tray impression
  - Single mix technique
  - Regular body or Monophase material.
- Closed bite double arch method or triple tray technique
- Copper tube/band impression
  - Low fusing compound.
- Post space impression
  - Light body
  - Wax.

Q. 62. What are the advantages of electroforming?

Ans. The advantages are as follows:

- They are stronger
- Have better marginal defination
- It is easier to wax and dewax a pattern several times
- Less injury to the cast, while finishing the casting
- Dimensionally stable
- Good abrassive resistance.

Q. 63. What is a metallizing agent? Name a few examples.

Ans. Metallizing agent is one which when applied on the surface of an impression, makes the surface conductable to current.

For examples:

- Bronze powder with oil of better almond colloidal silver in water—silver electroforming
- Finely powered silver or copper
- Aquadag which is a suspension of colloidal graphite in water copper electroforming.

Q. 64. What is a working model?

Ans. A working model die is the one from which dies can be removed.

The dies are single tooth replicas prepared for easier handling during wax pattern fabrication, and finishing of inaccessible areas of the cast.

Q. 65. What are the advantages of a working model?

Ans. The advantages of a working model are:

- To be able to remove the die and dip it in molten wax to get a close adaptation of wax
- To be able to get a good carving at the gingival finishing line
- To achieve a good contact point
- To be able to visualize a distoration in a casting.

Q. 66. What are the different investment materials?

Ans. The different investment materials are:

- Gypsum bonded investment—gold alloy
- Phosphate bonded investment—chrome cobalt—Withstand high temperature
- Silica bounded investment, this can be used in place of phosphate bonded investment.

Q. 67. What should be the length of the sprue?

Ans. The length of the sprue should be such that when the wax pattern is in the casting ring, it should be 1/4th of an inch away from the open end of the ring.

Q. 68. What is a reservoir?

Ans. A reservoir is one which acts a feeder of molten metal during casting. It is 1/16th away from the pattern. On the sprue, additional wax is added to thicken it or the sprue is fanned out at the point, it is joined with the pattern to acts as a reservoir.

This provides molten metal while metal in the mould solidifies thereby preventing shrinkage porosity during casting.

Q. 69. Why do you line the casting ring with ringliner?

Ans. The casting ring is lined with a ringliner to:

- Allow the effective setting and thermal expansion to take place
- Insulate against loss of heat during casting
- Facilitates the removal of the investment from the ring after casting is completed.

Q. 70. How would you compensate for the casting shrinkage of metal?

Ans. Shrinkage of metal can be compensated by:

- The setting expansion of the investment material
- Thermal expansion of the investment material
- Hygroscopic expansion of the investment material
- Preparing the die in type V gypsum which is a high strength high expansion gypsum material.

Q. 71. What type of a casting ring would you use for a hygroscopic investment material?

Ans. A split ring or a rubber ring is used for hygroscopic investment material.

Q. 72. What are ringless castings?

Ans. Ringless castings is the procedure in which no metal casting rings are used for investing the wax pattern. Paper or plastic rings are used which are removed after the investment sets. Ringless casting allows undisturbed expansion of the investment to take place.

Q. 73. What is pickling?

Ans. Pickling is a process to eliminate surface oxides in a gold casting. This is done by placing the casting in 40–50% solution of hydrogen chloride or/and bought to boiling point.

Q. 74. What are the casting defects?

Ans. The casting defects are:

- Dimensional inaccuracy
- Surface roughness
- Porosity
- Incomplete casting.

Q. 75. What is spot porosity or shrinkage porosity?

Ans. It is porosity caused when inadequate molten metal is available during solidification of metal in the mold. This is due to very thin sprue or no reservoir provided while spruing the wax pattern.

Q. 76. What is backpressure porosity?

Ans. This is caused by the inability of the air in the mold to escape through the pores of the investment or by the pressure gradient that displaces the air pocket towards the end of the investment via the molten sprue and button.

Its occurrence is reduced by:

- Using more porous investment
- Proper burnout
- Proper water powder ratio
- Adequate mold and casting temperature
- Sufficiently high casting pressure
- Locating the pattern near the end of the ring (6–8 mm).

Q. 77. What is soldering?

Ans. It is a process used to unite or bring into or restore to a firm union, the act of uniting two pieces of metal by the proper alloys of metals.

Q. 78. What is flux?

Ans. Any substance applied to surfaces to be joined by brazing, soldering or welding to clean and free them from oxides and promote union.

Q. 79. What are the different types of precision attachments?

Ans. The different types of precision attachments are as follows:

- Coronal
  - Extracoronal
  - Intracoronal
  - Circum-coronal.
- Radicular
- Interdental
- Any of the above additional screws or springs.

Q. 80. What are the types of pontics?

Ans. Pontics can be of the following types

- Depending on the contact of mucosal contact
  - With mucosal contact
    - Ridge lap pontic
    - Modified ridge lap pontic
    - Ovate pontic
    - Saddle pontic.
  - Without mucosal contact
    - Sanitary or hygienic pontic
    - Bullet pontic.

- Depending on the type of material used
  - Prefabricated pontic
    - ¤ Trupontic
    - ¤ Interchangeable facing
    - ¤ Sanitary pontic
    - ¤ Pin-facing pontic
    - ¤ Modified pin-facing pontic
    - ¤ Reverse pin-facing pontic
    - ¤ Harmony pontic
    - ¤ Porcelain fused to metal pontic.
  - Custom made pontic
  - Prefabricated custom modified pontic.
- Depending on the type of material used
  - Metal and porcelain veneered pontic
  - Metal and resin veneered pontic
  - All metal pontic
  - All ceramic pontic.

Q. 81. Which is the ideal material for a pontic?

Ans. In the anterior region porcelain in the posterior region porcelain fused metal/metal.

The gingival contact area should be made of highly glazed porcelain as it is best tolerated by the tissues.

Q. 82. How would you design the occlusal surfaces of a pontic?

Ans. The pontic should be narrow buccolingually and should have additional grooves which will facilitate the escape of food during mastication. At the same time, it should occlude with the natural tooth.

Q. 83. What is a laminate?

Ans. A laminate is a thin shell like covering on tooth surface either of ceramic, composite or modified composite where there is no change in the tooth color from the original tooth shade.

Q. 84. What is a veneer?

Ans. A thin shell like covering of ceramic, composite or modified composite where there is change in shade of tooth.

Q. 85. What is a laminate veneer?

Ans. Laminate veneer is a thin covering on the surface of tooth either ceramic, composite or modified composite (ceromers) to change the shape and shade of the natural tooth.

Q. 86. What are the materials used for laminate veneer?

Ans. Most commonly used materials for laminate veneer are porcelain, composites or ceromers.

Q. 87. What are the indications of laminate veneer?

Ans. Various indications of laminate veneer include:

- Enamel hypoplasia
- Tooth discoloration
- Intrinsic stain, such as tretracyline staining
- Fractured teeth
- Closure of diastema
- Correction of anatomically malformed anterior teeth
- Young patients.

Q. 88. What are the different types of partial veneers?

Ans. Partial veneers may be classified according to:

- Materials
  - Ceramic
  - Metal
  - Ceromer.

- Surface covred
  - Anterior : 3/4, lingual, labial with laminates
  - Posterior : 3/4, 7/8th, mesial half.

Q. 89. What are adhesive bridges?

Ans. Adhesive bridges are also known as resin bonded bridges. These prosthesis are luted to tooth structure primarily enamel, which has been etched to provide mechanical retention for the resin cement.

Q. 90. What are the indications of adhesive bridges?

Ans. Adhesive bridges are indicated in:

- Caries-free abutment teeth
- Maxillary and mandibular incisor replacement
- Periodontal splints.
- Single posterior tooth replacements.

Q. 91. What are the advantages of adhesive bridge?

Ans. Adhesive bridges have the following advantages:

- Noninvasive, decreased pulpal irritation
- Decreased gingival irritation due to supragingival finishing line
- Comfortable to the patient
- Reduced cost.

Q. 92. What are the different types of adhesive bridges?

Ans. Adhesive bridges are of following types:

1. Rochette bridge—macroretention
2. Maryland bridge—microretention
3. Virginia bridge—macroretention.

Q. 93. What are ceramics?

Ans. Ceramics are nonmetallic and inorganic material formed after baking at high temperature.

Q. 94. How are ceramics classified?

Ans. Ceramics are classified as follows:

- According to the firing temperature
  - High fusing
  - Medium fusing
  - Low fusing.
- According to use
  - Fabrication of artificial teeth
  - Fabrication of crowns and inlays
  - Fabrication of metal ceramic restorations.
- According to the method of firing
  - Air fired
  - Vacuum fired.
- According to application
  - Core porcelain
  - Dentine or body porcelain
  - Enamel porcelain
  - Glaze porcelain.

Q. 95. What are the different all ceramic system?

Ans. The different all ceramics systems used in dentistry are:

1. Conventional powder slurry ceramic—Optic HSP, Duceram
2. Infiltrated ceramic systems—Inceram, aluminous PJC
3. Castable ceramic system—Dicor, Cerapol
4. Pressable ceramic system—IPS Empress, Optec
5. Machinable ceramic system—Cerec, Celay Lava.

Q. 96. What are the glass modifiers used in porcelain?

Ans. Potassium, sodium and calcium oxides are the glass modifiers used in dental porcelain.

Q. 97. What is alumina reinforced porcelain?

Ans. It is a medium fusing porcelain with alumina oxide in 40–50% by volume. It has a high fracture strength. Fusion Temperature is 1950–2000°F.

Q. 98. What are the indications of metal ceramic restoration?

Ans. The indications of metal ceramic restoration are as follows:

- Teeth that require complete coverage in the esthetic zone
- Cases of extensive tooth destruction in the esthetic zone
- Need for superior retention and strength
- An endodontically treated tooth with post and core.

Q. 99. What features should be checked at the metal try-in stage?

Ans. At metal try- in stage, the following features should be checked.

- Marginal integrity
- Proximal contact
- Stability
- Occlusion.

Q. 100. What are metal-ceramic alloys?

Ans. Metal ceramic alloys are divided into:

- Noble metal alloys (or precious alloy)
  - Gold-platinum-palladium
  - Gold-palladium-silver
  - Gold-palladium
  - Palladium-silver
  - High palladium.

- Base metal alloys
  - Nickel-chromium
  - Cobalt-chromium.
- Other systems.

Q. 101. What are the different ways for shade selection?

Ans. Shade selection can be done:

- Visually
- Using shade guide
- Colorimeter
- Spectrophotometer.

Q. 102. What are the different shade guides?

Ans.
- VITA-Classic shade guide
- VITAPAN-3D Master shade guide.

Q. 103. What are the failures expected in fixed partial dentures?

Ans. Failures in fixed partial dentures can be due to:

- Cementation failure
- Mechanical break down of retainer, pontic or connector
- Gingival irritation
- P riodontal breakdown
- Caries
- Pulpal necrosis.

Q. 104. Which methods are applied to remove a fixed partial denture?

Ans. A fixed partial denture can be removed by the following methods:

- Using a crown remover
- By cutting the retainer with a bur
- Using an ultrasonic scaler tip
- Using a straight chisel
- Using a sticky crown remover.

Index

V

W

X

Y

Z